Philosophy of Population Health

Population health has recently grown from a series of loosely connected critiques of twentieth-century public health and medicine into a theoretical framework with a corresponding field of research—population health science. Its approach is to promote the public's health through improving everyday human life: affordable nutritious food, clean air, safe places where children can play, living wages, etc. It recognizes that addressing contemporary health challenges such as the prevalence of type 2 diabetes will take much more than good hospitals and public health departments.

Blending philosophy of science/medicine, public health ethics and history, *Philosophy of Population Health* offers a framework that explains, analyses and largely endorses the features that define this relatively new field. Presenting a philosophical perspective, Valles helps to clarify what these features are and why they matter, including: searching for health's "upstream" causes in social life, embracing a professional commitment to studying and ameliorating the staggering health inequities in and between populations; and reforming scientific practices to foster humility and respect among the many scientists and non-scientists who must work collaboratively to promote health.

Featuring illustrative case studies from around the globe at the end of all main chapters, this radical monograph is written to be accessible to all scholars and advanced students who have an interest in health—from public health students to professional philosophers.

Sean A. Valles is Associate Professor, jointly appointed to Michigan State University's Lyman Briggs College and Department of Philosophy, USA.

History and Philosophy of Biology

Series editor: Rasmus Grønfeldt Winther | rgw@ucsc.edu | www.rgwinther.com

This series explores significant developments in the life sciences from historical and philosophical perspectives. Historical episodes include Aristotelian biology, Greek and Islamic biology and medicine, Renaissance biology, natural history, Darwinian evolution, Nineteenth-century physiology and cell theory, Twentieth-century genetics, ecology, and systematics, and the biological theories and practices of non–Western perspectives. Philosophical topics include individuality, reductionism and holism, fitness, levels of selection, mechanism and teleology, and the nature–nurture debates, as well as explanation, confirmation, inference, experiment, scientific practice, and models and theories vis-à-vis the biological sciences.

Authors are also invited to inquire into the "and" of this series. How has, does, and will the history of biology impact philosophical understandings of life? How can philosophy help us analyze the historical contingency of, and structural constraints on, scientific knowledge about biological processes and systems? In probing the interweaving of history and philosophy of biology, scholarly investigation could usefully turn to values, power, and potential future uses and abuses of biological knowledge.

The scientific scope of the series includes evolutionary theory, environmental sciences, genomics, molecular biology, systems biology, biotechnology, biomedicine, race and ethnicity, and sex and gender. These areas of the biological sciences are not silos, and tracking their impact on other sciences such as psychology, economics, and sociology, and the behavioral and human sciences more generally, is also within the purview of this series.

Rasmus Grønfeldt Winther is Associate Professor of Philosophy at the University of California, Santa Cruz (UCSC), and Visiting Scholar of Philosophy at Stanford University (2015–2016). He works in the philosophy of science and philosophy of biology and has strong interests in metaphysics, epistemology, and political philosophy, in addition to cartography and GIS, cosmology and particle physics, psychological and cognitive science, and science in general. Recent publications include "The Structure of Scientific Theories," *The Stanford Encyclopaedia of Philosophy* and "Race and Biology," *The Routledge Companion to the Philosophy of Race*. His book with University of Chicago Press, *When Maps Become the World*, is forthcoming.

Philosophy of Population Health

Philosophy for a New Public Health Era

Sean A. Valles

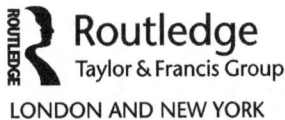

Routledge
Taylor & Francis Group

LONDON AND NEW YORK

First published 2018
by Routledge

2 Park Square, Milton Park, Abingdon, Oxfordshire OX14 4RN
52 Vanderbilt Avenue, New York, NY 10017

Routledge is an imprint of the Taylor & Francis Group, an informa business

First issued in paperback 2019

British Library Cataloguing in Publication Data
A catalogue record for this book is available from the British Library

Library of Congress Cataloging in Publication Data
Names: Valles, Sean A. (Sean Alejandro) author.
Title: Philosophy of population health science : philosophy for a new
public health era / Sean A. Valles.
Description: Milton Park, Abingdon, Oxon ; New York, NY : Routledge,
2018. | Includes bibliographical references and index.
Identifiers: LCCN 2017060479| ISBN 9781138059900 (hbk) |
ISBN 9781315163307 (ebk)
Subjects: LCSH: Social medicine–Philosophy. | Medicine–Philosophy.
Classification: LCC RA418 .V357 2018 | DDC 362.1–dc23
LC record available at https://lccn.loc.gov/2017060479

ISBN: 978-1-138-05990-0 (hbk)
ISBN: 978-0-367-35862-4 (pbk)

Typeset in Times New Roman
by Wearset Ltd, Boldon, Tyne and Wear

A tu salud, Maya.

Contents

Illustrations

Acknowledgments

Thanks go first and foremost to Margot Valles, for the constant and patient support throughout the writing of this book.

I owe great thanks to Elizabeth Simmons, Matt McKeon, and Chris Long for making my sabbatical possible and hence making the writing of this book possible.

I have been greatly assisted at various writing stages with text feedback from: Robyn Bluhm, Anke Bueter, Teresa Blankmeyer Burke, Laura Cabrera, Kristie Dotson, Kevin Elliott, Sandro Galea, Kerry Keyes, Shelbi Meissner, Nancy McHugh, David Nash, Billy Oglesby, Alexandria Skoufalos, Dan Steel, and Kyle Whyte.

For their questions and comments, I thank the attendees of: the Nov. 2016 Philosophy of Science Association; the Dec. 2016 Michigan State University Department of Philosophy colloquium; the Mar. 2017 Wittenberg University colloquium; the Apr. 2017 American Philosophical Association—Pacific Division; the Jun. 2017 International Philosophy of Medicine Roundtable; the Aug. 2017 Massey University Diversity in Philosophy Conference, the incarcerated and non-incarcerated students in the spring 2017 Wittenberg University course "Global Health Justice"; and the students of the fall 2017 Michigan State University course, "Introduction to Science, Technology, the Environment and Public Policy."

For starting me down this path, I thank the Edinburgh Migration, Ethnicity, and Health Research Group, the University of Edinburgh Centre for Population Health Sciences, and especially Raj Bhopal and Vittal Katikireddi.

I thank my parents, Marilyn Valles and Larry Valles, for their even earlier efforts at setting me on a life course trajectory of well-being—I owe my life course thinking to their life course efforts.

All remaining mistakes in the book are my own.

1 Blueprint of a philosophy of—and for—population health

A brief overview

This book offers a detailed philosophical analysis of the features and consequences of the emerging "population health science" and associated population health "approach"/"framework"/"thinking." Population health is a bold intellectual and practical expansion of "public health." The corresponding population health science synthesizes expertise from an array of scientists and nonscientists to understand the full range of causes of health and illness in a population (from gun violence to food affordability), seeking to improve health through collaborations between multiple sectors of society (from insurance companies to community activists). It is now widely accepted that effective and equitable health promotion requires broad-scoped interdisciplinary and intersectoral efforts. Accordingly, use of the term "population health" is growing exponentially in publications, and the term is getting incorporated into the names and/ or missions of colleges, departments, centers, and academic journals worldwide. Yet, no previous philosophy book has offered a concerted analysis of the rise of the population health science. This book fills the gap, seeking to contribute to both the philosophy community (which too often critiques an outdated notion of public health) and the population health community, which has grown so quickly that it is inevitably still sorting through its assumptions, theories, values: what they are, what they could be, and what they should be.

The book begins by articulating the history of population health science, rooted in the gradual recognition of health as a social phenomenon. Next, the book argues for a pluralistic understanding of health as something inherently tied to the nuances of diverse social contexts and necessarily understood as something extended over the entire life course; this is offered as a meta-concept of health that leaves room for a plurality of locally contingent healths. The following chapter argues that population health science offers a way to expand public health's scope of interests and interventions, while still respecting philosophers' concerns about public health becoming hegemonic. Broad models of public/population health such as "health in all policies," seek to promote population health via action on social and environmental determinants of health (e.g., tax reforms to address economic inequities), but overtly reject the notion that physicians or public health officials should dictate social policy from on high. The next chapter argues that attending to philosophy of causation in population health indicates the need for special attention to health's "upstream causes" (including so-called "fundamental causes") and their downstream effects, with an eye toward explaining the causes of massive health disparities between populations. The next chapter identifies some key enduring methodological challenges, including how population health science research and interventions struggle with questions about how to proceed in the absence of abundant evidence from randomized controlled trials, and how to divide up populations in order to examine and intervene upon the needs of various subpopulations. The following chapter argues that health equity concerns are inseparable from the practice of population health science, but that the philosophical and conceptual obstacles to promoting health equity need to be reappraised. Lack of consensus about the meaning and moral justification of health equity are manageable inevitabilities, while relatively more attention is owed to advancing health equity by first creating inclusive and participatory decision-making processes. The final chapter reiterates the cross-cutting importance of epistemic humility: we each need to recognize our limitations as knowers, and moving forward in population health science requires humble and non-hierarchical collaborative relationships—intersectoral and interdisciplinary. Moreover, the relatively small group of scholars who are familiar with population health science have an obligation to communicate with the public about what population health science is and does.

Introduction

Public health isn't what it used to be; sometimes it's not even "public health"— it's "population health." This book is a philosophical take on the rise of "population health," which is has become ubiquitous over the last two decades, yet remains unknown to all but a small group of health scholars and practitioners. Since the 1990s, a growing number of public health scholars, practitioners, and policymakers have begun using the term "population health." This curious term signals growing support for a new set of theories and methods—those of population health as opposed to a narrowly conceived public health. The population health literature is heterogeneous, but at its core is a set of radical and admirable new ideas about how to reform the way we promote healthy populations. These ideas have been described and debated, largely in fragmentary articles, accompanied by a handful of science books attempting to synthesize together what it means to adopt a population health approach/thinking/model/paradigm and what it means to do applied science under the aegis of "population health." Meanwhile, philosophers specializing in the public health sciences have done little to aid in the project of analyzing, synthesizing, and communicating what is philosophically novel or notable about the shift that is signified by the phrase "population health." This book seeks to help remedy that gap in the literature by constructing a philosophical scaffold to intellectually support population health science. This book shows how population health science's fragmentary theoretical and methodological pieces do indeed fit together, and that the complete interdisciplinary whole they assemble is well positioned to change for the better the theory and practice of health promotion.

A clear understanding of philosophical questions in population health—from how to define health and conceptualize causes, to how health equity values fit into the practice of population health—can contribute to future debates over what it does mean and what it should mean to work in the service of "population health." Overall, this is a book that hopes to make some small contribution to the population health project—it is philosophy *of* population health in the form of philosophy *for* population health—with the long-term goal of advancing population health science and expanding the dialogue between philosophy and population health science. To do this, the book will integrate philosophy of science, philosophy of medicine, bioethics, and public health ethics.

Philosophers of science and medicine, like me, spend a great deal of time examining the philosophical foundations of sprawling disciplines/theories/enterprises, small projects/hypotheses/texts, and everything between. Much like building inspectors or health inspectors, we typically find a combination of individually avoidable errors, dubious shortcuts, and ill-designed methods. All the while, philosophers of science and medicine still tend to have an abiding respect and appreciation for science/medicine, critiquing in the hopes of making things better. When scrutinizing the philosophical underpinnings of a new interdisciplinary program (such as in my previous work on evolutionary medicine and personalized genomic medicine), I have come to expect extensive, if not fatal, problems (Valles 2012a; Valles 2012b). Imagine my surprise at encountering population health science and finding nothing really fundamentally broken. What I found instead was a field that has many debates and unsettled theoretical and practical questions that remain to be sorted out, and many open questions about the future of the field. So, I come to this project on philosophy of population health science as a philosopher of science and medicine seeing little broken in the field, but still seeing many questions—about what population health science is, was, should be, and could be—that I think my skill set can help answer or at least clarify. I see population health science as a thoughtful reaction by public health scientists and other health scientists, a reaction against practices that had proliferated in twentieth-century biomedical science and influenced much of public health science: the paternalism, the overreliance on narrow biomedical understandings of health and well-being, the cultural and ethical imperialism, the failures to connect with underlying social problems such as food insecurity, the arrogance of expert judgments delivered by experts from on high.

Philosopher of biology Michael Ruse has pondered whether philosophy of science should take up the role of "handmaiden to the sciences" (Ruse 2008). I prefer the framing offered by Kristie Dotson, who has advocated for philosophy done from a "position of service" (Dotson 2015). So, I offer this book from a position of service to scholars and graduate/professional students interested in population health—philosophers and non-philosophers alike.

What is population health science?

Population health science is a loosely organized field of research and practice, united by a commitment to understanding patterns of health distribution within and between human populations, and to achieving desirable equitable patterns of health distribution via interdisciplinary and intersectoral efforts. It is also committed to the view that health's causes and effects are embedded in nuanced ways within human populations' diverse cultures, social structures, and environments. Population health science is pluralistic in the sense that it seeks those interdisciplinary and intersectoral collaborations because they are theoretically irreplaceable, not just expedient. Population health science is sprawling in scope to match its contention that health is similarly massive. Neither sociology nor epidemiology can have a suitably complete grasp of health; neither patient advocacy charities nor for-profit healthcare companies can fully succeed in promoting health without the cooperation of the other. There are entrenched antagonisms impeding these sorts of interdisciplinary and intersectoral collaborations, but this does nothing to dissuade population health science advocates from the belief that we nonetheless need such collaborations.

Population health science is in the early formative stages of a new discipline. Right now, population health science "represents a way of thinking, rather than a particular set of questions or methods and, as such, draws from a number of long-standing disciplines" (Keyes and Galea 2016b: 633). Population health science scholars have offered varying, but complementary, definitions for what "population health" signifies as a practical scientific enterprise:

> a conceptual approach to understanding the drivers of health and consequently the strategies most useful to improve health. As I see it, this conceptual approach has two key principles: (1) the need to consider factors defined at multiple levels of organization … and (2) an explicit concern with health equity.
>
> (Diez Roux 2016)

> the field of population health includes health outcomes, patterns of health determinants, and policies and interventions that link these two.
>
> (Kindig and Stoddart 2003: 380)

> a research program that confronts the structural forces that place individuals at risk, creates distributions of health and disease unequally across socially defined groups, and focuses on embedding biological pathways within social interactions that develop across the life course and across generations.
>
> (Keyes and Galea 2016b: 634)

> population health connects prevention, wellness, and behavioral health science with healthcare quality and safety, disease prevention, and management and economic issues of value and risk—all in the service of the specific population.
>
> (Nash et al. 2016: xviii)

population health has a focus on health disparities, particularly disparities related to socioeconomic status, and many of its proponents have a pessimistic view of the degree to which health care can reduce these disparities.

(Anderson et al. 2005: 757)

This book will proceed under my reading of what falls under the broad population health science framework, which I interpret as: (1) rooted in theoretical and empirical developments in the mid-late twentieth century (Marmot et al. 1984; Rose 1992); (2) shaped by World Health Organization priority-setting (World Health Organization 1986; Commission on Social Determinants of Health 2008; Kickbusch 2003; Murray et al. 2002; World Health Organization 2014); (3) spurred by the 1994 volume *Why Are Some People Healthy and Others Not?* (Evans et al. 1994); (4) popularized by Kindig and Stoddart (Kindig and Stoddart 2003; Kindig 2007); (5) heralded by the growth of departments/colleges/centers of "population health" (Bachrach et al. 2015); (6) pursued under various names and models in contemporary work, often using the term "population health" (Tricco et al. 2008; Stoto 2013); and (7) summarized in a handful of general texts (Young 1998; Keyes and Galea 2016a; Nash et al. 2016). The lingering fogginess of what does and doesn't fall within this interdisciplinary endeavor (Tricco et al. 2008; Jacobson and Teutsch 2012) is one of the chief motivations for my writing this book.

In this book I will use the term "population health science" to refer to the scientific dimension of the larger "population health framework." Advocates of population health science tend to agree that it "represents a way of thinking (Keyes and Galea 2016b: 633)," one that is not restricted to scientists or even scientific reasoning—there is more to a population health *framework* than population health *science*. For example, the population health framework is concerned with instilling new population health thinking in people such as employers, so that they can appreciate and address the ways that employees' wellness is good for all parties (Isaac and Gorhan 2016). I prefer "population health framework" as the descriptor for the umbrella way of thinking, including population health science. This is in keeping with a key article in the development of population health—"Why Population Health?" by John Frank (Frank 1995) and some subsequent literature, including work on population health terminology by David Kindig, one of the leading contemporary scholars on the topic (Kindig 2007). However, others refer to it as the "population health model," which is a misnomer due to the diffuse theoretical and practical commitments of population health scholars (Carpiano and Daley 2006), and because the "Population Health Model" ("POHEM") is a particular microsimulation computer model developed by early population health science scholars in Canada, a model which only a small subset in population health work uses (Hennessy et al. 2015).

The upcoming chapters will strive for clarity in their use of key and often related terms, such as "population health" and "public health." The trickiness of these terminological questions is largely a reflection of the field itself. Even the term "population health" is a known source of confusion since it is used in the literature to refer to both the phenomenon itself and the corresponding field of study (Nash et al. 2016: 3; Kindig and Stoddart 2003). Confusion over the meaning of "population health" has also affected the (small) philosophical literature on it. Rothstein has attacked the creeping of "population health" theories and practices into the domain of "public health," while Goldberg has sometimes defended "population health" under the label "broad model of public health" (Rothstein 2002, 2009; Goldberg 2012). Exasperated at the terminological confusions, Diez Roux insists that Goldberg's use of the term "public health" is identical to how advocates use the term "population health" (Diez Roux 2016); DeSalvo splits the difference by proposing the term "Public Health 3.0" (DeSalvo et al. 2016). And so on.

Terminological disputes are typical in young and developing fields. In spite of the field's youth, population health science's tenets have already had enormous success in mainstream public health. This is in keeping with an ambition to reform, expand, and reorient public health science, rather than to reject and compete with public health. It has found a particularly warm reception in the American Public Health Association, which hosts the world's largest annual public health conference. It is telling (and rhetorically convenient) that APHA's recent conference themes, when combined, serve as a thumbnail sketch of key components of a sound philosophical foundation for population health science:

- Health is a social entity, and health promotion must also be social (Chapter 2)

  - "Healthy Communities Promote Healthy Minds and Bodies" (2011 American Public Health Association conference theme)

- Health is a life course phenomenon, and best approached as such (Chapter 3)

  - "Prevention and Wellness Across The Life Span" (2012 American Public Health Association conference theme)

- Health promotion efforts must be willing to contend with the massive breadth of health's socially embedded causes and effects (Chapters 4 and 5)

  - "Think Global, Act Local" (2013 American Public Health Association conference theme)
  - "Healthography: How Where You Live Affects Your Health and Well-Being" (2014 American Public Health Association conference theme)
  - "Health in all Policies" (2015 American Public Health Association conference theme)

- Social justice and social reform are necessary components of population health promotion, even if achieving this will be difficult and contentious (Chapters 6 and 7)

- "Social Justice: A Public Health Imperative" (2010 American Public Health Association conference theme)
- "Creating the Healthiest Nation: Ensuring the Right to Health" (2016 American Public Health Association conference theme)

Meanwhile, the 2016 accrediting standards for US public health higher education programs make frequent reference to "population health" (a change from the 2011 standards, which did not), including the requirement that Masters-level and Doctoral-level education must, "substantively address scientific and analytic approaches to discovery and translation of public health knowledge in the context of a population health framework" (Council on Education for Public Health 2016: 29). Population health science is a distinct entity at this point, but some readers will recognize similarities with kindred disciplines and movements. Social medicine and the People's Health Movement are two such endeavors. Interestingly, despite many similarities between population health science and these other two entities, the practical relationships between them are far weaker than one might expect. They share the commonality of having developed as reactions against undesirable features of the biomedical model of health, which dominated the twentieth century (see Chapter 2). Chapter 6 will go on to show how evidence-based medicine is yet another field/movement that shares this dissatisfaction with the biomedical model, though evidence-based medicine's focus on healthcare interventions, and relative neglect of health promotion efforts outside the healthcare sector (in part because such interventions can be harder to assess), has led to peculiar tensions between it and population health science.

Perhaps the best illustration of the gap between the population health science and Social Medicine is that the term "Social Medicine" does not even appear in Nash et al.'s 2016 second edition to their population health textbook (Nash et al. 2016). The term appears exactly once in Keyes and Galea's book articulating population health science theory—in the MESH standardized medical keywords, "Social Medicine—methods" classifying the book's subjects; it appears nowhere in the text. Why the divergence of "population health" and "social medicine"? There are innumerable structural and disciplinary contingencies that surely played a role, but there is more essential philosophical reason at the heart of the disagreement. As Young argues in his population health text, "social medicine" and "preventive medicine" necessarily fall within the medical profession, and "social medicine" remains a liability for three reasons: (1) philosophically, it is tied to a "'biomedical' orientation" that is fundamentally objectionable to the many skeptics of the biomedical model of population health promotion (even if social medicine pushes back against biomedicalization); (2) "social medicine" can be confused with the politically contentious "socialized" medicine (though Chapter 2 will argue that the connections to socialism are more than an accident of terminology); and (3) "proponents of population health" have situated themselves as offering "something more than traditional public health" (Young 2005: 5).

Why write a book on philosophy of population health science?

Population health science has made enormous strides, and philosophers have much work to do to catch up. While this book will make clear that I largely endorse the trajectory of population health science, the lack of public awareness that there even is such a thing, let alone its previous and potential accomplishments, is deeply problematic. This book is offering a small contribution to meeting that need by working to build a critical dialogue around the many philosophical aspects of population health science. Critical dialogue is very much in the spirit of population health science since, historically, the field is the result of public health scientists coming to terms with internal and external criticism. Chapter 2 chronicles that process in detail, but the point for the moment is that population health scientists have echoed scholars' critiques about how public health needed a course correction—population health science is a field of science devoted to doing this. In the 1994 edited volume that arguably marks the birth of population health science, Renaud metaphorically described the fundamental tension as a power struggle between Panakeia, the goddess of medicine (individualistic biomedical thinking) and Hygeia, the goddess of public health (population thinking):

> On the eve of the twenty-first century, a power struggle emerges between the god of medical art, Panakeia, who is increasingly ambitious and skillful in her attempts to resurrect the dead, and Hygeia, the goddess of public health and great priestess of social reforms.
>
> (Renaud 1994: 324)

> In the realm of health, the issue at stake for the future is the reestablishment of a balance between Hygeia and Panakeia, which has been tilted in favour of the latter over the course of three decades of biomedical development.
>
> (Renaud 1994: 333)

Renaud was correct in his era about the problem of patient-level care displacing population-level health, and hindsight makes it look all the more prophetic of him to contribute to a whole new field of science to address the problem.

Public health science has come under frequent attack by a number of philosophers, anthropologists, and other humanists and social scientists studying it. The tension between individualistic biomedicine and population-level health matters is responsible for many of the critiques of public health coming from scholars and laypeople alike. To name a few focal problems:

*   A slew of behavioral guidelines relentlessly add new behavioral expectations for individuals, adding up to an absurdly untenable and inappropriate burden for each person.

    *   "Lose weight!" "Avoid fat!" "Stop smoking!" "Reduce alcohol intake!" "Get fit!" "Practice safe sex!" "Play safe!" ... Individuals are expected

to take responsibility for the care of their bodies and to limit their potential to harm others through taking up various preventive actions.

(Petersen and Lupton 1996: ix)

- Public health science is all too often wielded bluntly, without due attention to the fact that evidentiary/epistemic and ethical/values standards for public health experts are often very different from those of the populations they try to serve.

  - While parents and public health officials may hold many values in common, their value hierarchies are sometimes at odds, and the rules by which they wage arguments often differ considerably. The result is a chaotic environment in which, parents ... ultimately decide whether or not to vaccinate children.

    (Largent 2012: 29)

- Even seemingly benign concepts and theoretical innovations in public health science have combined to elevate individual lifestyle and risk factors, at the expense of other understandings of what population-level health is and how its causes are approached.

  - New methods and approaches for studying health, a shift from earlier mechanistic approaches to probabilistic lifestyle factors, and the rise of "chronic disease," evolved synergistically to converge in an emphasis on lifestyle as a core—really, *the* core—problem confronting public health.

    (Bell 2017: 26)

I agree that these are genuine and serious problems. And the problems go much further. The dominant biomedical model of health—elaborated in Chapter 2—with its focus on disease, diagnosis and bio-technological patient-level solutions to population-level problems, has been a massive disappointment despite massive social investments in it. Bell's text *Health and Other Unassailable Values* (Bell 2017) and Metzl and Kirkland's volume *Against Health* (Metzl and Kirkland 2010) together offer detailed and insightful analysis of the often moralistic follies that can and do creep into public health science literature and the associated public/media discourse. I support population health science in part *because* I take these criticisms of public health science very seriously. More importantly, I believe that the problems are already being addressed.

Medical science done under an implicit or explicit biomedical model has left a legacy of over-prescription (Welch et al. 2011), disease mongering (González-Moreno et al. 2015), profiteering (Goldacre 2012), and more. A burgeoning body of evidence indicates that the biomedical model is not just yielding the aforementioned side effects—it is arguably failing outright. The signs of this are appearing most conspicuously in my home country, the United States, where the biomedical model has long found fertile ground thanks to its research infrastructure, remarkable willingness to spend disproportionate amounts of its vast wealth on healthcare, and its reliance on novel medical treatments to address its health ills. Perhaps the most striking example of the model's failures are the data on the failures of the annual checkup—the exemplar of the biomedical model's contributions to routine population health monitoring and wellness, a hazily defined practice of scrutinizing a patient's vital signs and diagnostic tests in search of pathologies in patients' tissues. A meta-analysis of longitudinal studies that included a total of 182,800 subjects finds that annual checkups reduce neither morbidity nor mortality (Krogsbøll et al. 2012). Checkups' chief accomplishment is that they do in fact increase the number of diagnoses for patients (Krogsbøll et al. 2012)—the biomedical model is certainly good at making business for itself. In total, the sprawling US biomedical system is exorbitantly expensive and yet, by most measures, it yields abysmal results (Woolf and Aron 2013).

The good news is that the reform effort—population health science—already has a firm foothold and is making more headway all the time. Figure 1.1 is a variation on a diagram Sandro Galea previously published, in which he shows that 2013 marked a sudden change in the ratio of English-language PubMed database entries mentioning "population health science" divided by those mentioning "epidemiology"; 2013 was when ratio suddenly began exponentially climbing (Galea 2017). Figure 1.1 takes a similar approach and shows how in a little over 20 years, "population health" went from being a virtual non-entity to being used about 1/10 as often as "public health." A 1:10 ratio remains small, but three factors must be kept in mind. First, the "public health" phrase has been part of the health lexicon for over a century, appearing in academic journal names, institutions, professional titles (MPH, Master of Public Health), and everyday usage (the standard term for the health of a group of people is "public health"). Second, the increasing ratio means that "population health" is making gains *relative to* "public health"—"public health" and "population health" are

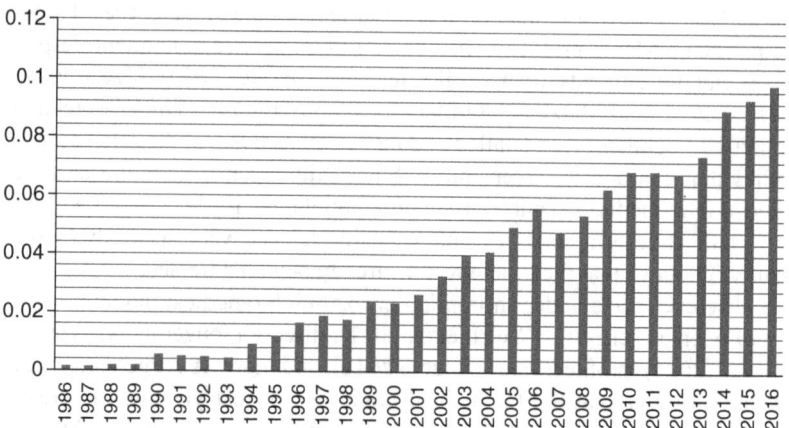

Figure 1.1 Ratio of the number of results from a PubMed search using "population health" as a search term divided by the number of results using "public health" as a search term, 1986–2016.

both used very often in health publications, but the growth of "population health" is outpacing "public health." Third, as noted above, population health science's impact is not just evidenced by invocations of the term; it has also made an enormous impact on public health science, such that some scholars see it as just good public health science (Diez Roux 2016), and others describe the contributions as a distinct new phase of public health science (DeSalvo et al. 2016).

There is clearly something happening in the public/population health sciences, something that merits attention. The rise of population health thinking is better tracked in the US and Canada than elsewhere—a sampling problem afflicting most areas of health research—but the data from the US are telling, and important insofar as the US and Canada together produce a large proportion of health science (the majority of it, according to a 2008 bibliometric analysis; Tricco et al. 2008). A 2015 report commissioned by the Institute of Medicine Roundtable on Population Health Improvement found 25 Masters- and/or PhD-level programs in the US including "population health" in their names (Bachrach et al. 2015). A survey of US hospitals by the American Hospital Association found, "over 90% of hospitals agreed or strongly agreed that population health was aligned with their mission" (Health Research & Educational Trust 2015: 4). With that degree of institutional entrenchment, it will not be going away anytime soon. The incredible power of institutional inertia and the impossibility of 'unringing the bell' after exposing students, administrators, etc. to population health thinking, means that this mindset will linger and echo for a long time, even if population health science were to start falling into decline for some reason.

Katherine Keyes and Sandro Galea's 2016 book, *Population Health Science*, lays out the theoretical scientific foundations of the contemporary population health sciences, and in doing so ends up engaging with some of the same questions addressed in this book (Keyes and Galea 2016a). Though, as an exposition of the general theoretical background of population health sciences, it is only able to engage in a limited way with most philosophical issues. For example, the book posits the "principle": "Efforts to improve overall population health may be a disadvantage to some groups; whether equity or efficiency is preferable is a matter of values" (Keyes and Galea 2016a). The book's need to get through a wide survey of the technical details of the science means that it cannot devote as much time to directly covering philosophical angles. Ultimately, I see my book as complementary to theirs; *Population Health Science* lays out the scientific foundations of population health science with some related discussion of philosophical matters, while this book lays out the philosophical matters with some related discussion of population health science.

Other works have also explored the gray areas between population health science theory and philosophy of population health science. For a textbook-type overview, the clear leader is Nash et al.'s updated textbook, which also includes thoughtful discussion of philosophical issues such as equity, overarching evidentiary/epistemic challenges, and political theoretical aspects of health promotion and governance (Nash et al. 2016). In 2002, the World Health Organization

(WHO) published an edited volume that served to foster conversation among the diffuse considerations and disciplines involved in population health measurement, including the ethical issues therein (Murray et al. 2002); though, edited volumes lack the sort of univocal cohesion of works such as T. Kue Young's monograph *Population Health: Concepts and Methods*, which had appeared four years earlier and includes discussion of philosophical issues such as the nature and measurement of health (Young 1998).

What will this book accomplish?

Chapter 2 historically traces population health science to a series of twentieth-century insights about the social nature of health:

> the recent "bio-medicalized" view, ascendant since the Flexner reform of North American medical schools ... focuses our attention, for example in coronary disease prevention, on the control of intermediary physiological variables, such as blood pressure, rather than the living and working conditions that may underlie their perturbation.
>
> (Frank 1995: 163)

The chapter traces out the twentieth-century history of how population health science emerged a new interdisciplinary approach. I argue that the history of population health science theory is best understood as the synthesis of four different insights that took hold in public health theory in the twentieth century: (1) health is metaphysically social, (2) health is empirically social, (3) health is ethically inseparable from social empowerment, and (4) methodologies of health research and health promotion must engage with health as a social phenomenon. The WHO, boldly and controversially, declared that health is the presence of complete well-being, including social well-being (World Health Organization 1946). It was not until the 1970s and 1980s that new data emerged to solidify the case that individuals' and populations' health are causally determined by social forces to an enormous degree. I trace the progression from this empirical data to the World Health Organization's dual embrace of health empowerment: empowering individuals and their communities is pragmatically essential according to emerging data on the social science of health, and also health empowerment is ethically essential as a means of promoting population health without committing paternalistic abuses. This commitment to empowerment spurred the development of new methodologies of research and intervention when interacting with populations during health promotion efforts.

This chapter links to the following chapter on the definition of health, by illustrating how the four senses of health-as-social combine to yield a strong rebuttal to the influential biomedical understanding of health and disease. The biomedical model of health sees health as the absence of some distinct malfunction in the body's machinery. It is a view that is widely embraced inside and outside medical research communities, and Christopher Boorse has, most prominently, expounded it as a philosophical position. This understanding of health does not entirely preclude pursuit of population health science efforts. For example, Norman Daniels endorses Boorse's view and yet also shares population health sciences' interest in intervening on the social determinants of health (Daniels 2008: 37). Yet, the history provided in this chapter shows that a biomedical understanding of health led health sciences astray in the twentieth century, and population health science arose from within the community of health scientists to try to reform the theory and practice of health science at the population level. The biomedical model's dominance in the twentieth century fostered the development of new blood tests, imaging technologies, surgical techniques, drugs, and devices. Yet, perhaps most emblematically, the United States is a global leader in medical technology innovations and medical education, but the existence of such technologies and experts has failed to prevent the national life expectancy from stagnating and recently even declining (Xu et al. 2016). The chapter illustrates the value of understanding health in the four senses of social through a case study on the health of the Standing Rock Sioux population in the United States. The case study examines the tribe's opposition to the Dakota Access Pipeline that traverses land that is vital to the well-being of the tribe. I show that the social understanding of health that I endorse allows a more thorough account of the health harms at stake.

Chapter 3 offers an (pluralistic) overarching concept of health: health as a life course trajectory of complete well-being in social context:

> binary views [of "individual versus population health"] … fail to use the rich information and interpretations that stem from a more comprehensive approach to health over the life course (i) of the individual within the collective and (ii) of the collective of interacting individuals.
>
> (Arah 2009: 242)

The metaphysical and epistemic significance of "health" and "disease" are vigorously debated in the philosophy of medicine literature (Carel and Cooper 2014). In this chapter, I offer a new definition of health that synthesizes together some of Onyebuchi Arah's insights into philosophy of population health science and the World Health Organization's enduring endorsement of health as the positive presence of well-being. Arah's conception of individual and population-level health partly built on earlier work by McDowell et al. (Arah 2009; McDowell et al. 2004). Arah characterizes health as a dynamical life course phenomenon, a developing thing that is extended over time and shaped by a complex set of factors from genetics to social conditions; such a thing must be understood and addressed in light of its complete trajectory and not snapshots in time (e.g., one's vital signs at the time of a single visit to the doctor). I also argue for the adoption of the oft-maligned WHO concept of health as the presence of holistic well-being, a definition that has been criticized as vague or mistaken by many scholars (including some population health science scholars). I argue that it is an outline of a definition, capable of being further specified in individual applications, not a fully developed definition that is ready to operationalize as is. It is more toolbox than tool. I argue for one particular specification of the WHO definition, combining it with the life course concept to yield health as a *lifelong* complete physical, mental and social well-being.

After offering my new health concept as a slight variation on the WHO concept, I argue that the concept, *health as a life course trajectory of complete well-being in social context*, strikes the right balance between empirically informed specificity and pluralism. As illustrated in the preceding chapter, health is social and hence socially contingent. This concept of health insists that health cannot be adequately understood as a phenomenon that exists at a single moment in time, but it necessarily refrains from dictating to any population what it means to have complete well-being. This final point is demonstrated in more detail in the chapter's case study, on efforts to promote the health of Aboriginal Australians and efforts within the context of colonial settler–indigenous power dynamics.

Chapter 4 defuses the public health "boundary problem"—the fear that public health could exceed its proper disciplinary and sociopolitical boundaries and thereby cause negative repercussions:

> We understand that health equity is a shared responsibility and requires the engagement of all sectors of government, of all segments of society, and of all members of the international community, in an "all for equity" and "health for all" global action.
>
> (World Health Organization 2011)

There is a troubling tension between the philosophical commitments of public/population health scientists and philosophers of public health. On one hand, many philosophers vehemently insist that we must mind the "boundary problem" of carefully delineating and policing the boundary line that constrains what can be properly treated as a public/population health problem (see, for example, Powers and Faden 2006; Broadbent 2013). On the other hand, public/population health scientists have now widely endorsed the idea that we must promote "Health in All Policies" (McQueen et al. 2012; Rudolph et al. 2013). Philosophers have adopted their position out of fears of potential negative repercussions of allowing scholars to public health-ify social problems such as crime and poor housing (Rothstein 2009). I argue that population health science is philosophically on the right track by searching the entire structure of society, not just healthcare and other obvious places, for the causes, effects, and solutions of health and disease. Empirically, it has long been clear that all manner of social dynamics are intimately causally connected to health, and healthcare only contributes to some (Lalonde 1974; Black et al. 1980). Health matters and healthcare matters are not coextensive, nor are physicians the automatic rightful leaders in addressing health matters.

I argue that attempts to limit the scope of public health investigation or action rest on three related missteps. First, much philosophy of public health works under the unnecessarily restrictive political philosophy conception of public health action as the expression of government power over the polity. This is already a narrow framing of what public health is or can be, but such a view is wholly inadequate for understanding the growth of population health science, since population health is founded on a commitment to the idea that promoting the health of populations requires collaborations between different sectors of society—governments, charities, informal community activist groups, etc.—and government is just one sector among co-equals. Second, I argue that concerns about public health growing hegemonic and overtaking all discourse about population health are mistaken. Some make the conceptual mistake of assuming that treating a problem (e.g., gun violence) as a health problem then implies it is *only* a health problem (e.g., gun violence is also a legal problem). Others make the mistake of speculating about the potential harms of a broad conception of public health (one that addresses problems such as firearm policy) instead of looking at the decades-long history of clearly positive effects of implementing such a conception collaboratively and intersectorally.

I conclude that we do not know the full range of potential risks and benefits of adopting a broad model of population health, attention to the full range of risks at stake ("inductive risks" and other "epistemic risks"), and a broad model is preferable partly in light of our limited knowledge. The chapter's case study illustrates the importance of a broad model of population health by exploring the work done, and work not yet done, on the population health aspects of global climate change.

Chapter 5 argues for how and why population health science should carry out its agenda to research and respond to the "upstream" social causes of health:

> social factors such as socioeconomic status and social support are likely "fundamental causes" of disease that, because they embody access to important resources, affect multiple disease outcomes through multiple mechanisms, and consequently maintain an association with disease even when intervening mechanisms change.
>
> (Link and Phelan 1995: 80)

Health, as argued in Chapter 3, is a dynamic process that develops over the course of one's lifetime, not just a switch that flips off and on when one falls ill with a diagnosable disease and then recovers from it (Commission on Social Determinants of Health 2008; Hertzman et al. 1994). Similarly, a network of "social determinants" serve as extraordinarily powerful causal factors in shaping our health (Marmot 2004). Contending with these and other lessons of twentieth-century public health spurred the growth of new models for understanding and intervening upon the "upstream" causes of ill health—factors such as poverty and racism that lead to many ill effects downstream. I argue that one particularly philosophically and practically important contribution to this effort is Link and Phelan's theory of "fundamental causes," described in the above quote (Link and

Phelan 1995). Unfortunately, the term "fundamental cause" gives a misleading characterization of what is causally unique—and uniquely valuable—about fundamental causes. Drawing upon work on the philosophy of causation, I show how fundamental causes are special because they manifest a unique sort of stability. Fundamental causes are stable in the direction of their effect on health (e.g., social stigma harms health) but the proximate mechanisms and the specific health effects vary enormously, depending on context. This creates a situation where we can promote health via addressing stigma even without fully knowing the mechanisms of how certain upstream causes operate or even all the ways that they harm health.

I proceed to contrast population health science's laudable attention to social determinants of health and upstream causes of health with Broadbent's less prominent coverage of these topics in his influential text *Philosophy of Epidemiology* (Broadbent 2013). I use Geoffrey Rose's distinction between causes of individual cases of disease vs. causes of between-population disease disparities to show that Broadbent's philosophy prioritizes the former types of cause while population health science prioritizes the latter type of cause (Rose 1992). I conclude by advocating for orienting philosophy of public/population health to the topic of salutogenesis rather than pathogenesis; the philosophical study of disease can easily crowd out attention to the philosophical study of health. I illustrate these recommended changes in how to approach health causation by examining Brazil's evolving HIV/AIDS policies.

Chapter 6 identifies four key philosophically rooted practical challenges faced by population health science:

> ideally, we want population health interventions that are both efficient and equitable. In many ways, however, these two goals—equity and efficiency—are often at odds with each other; that is, there is a tradeoff when maximizing one potentially results in a cost for the other.
>
> (Keyes and Galea 2016a: 130)

Applied population health science requires contending with difficult methodological choices along the way to achieving "health for all" (Fielding et al. 2013). In this chapter I make a case for why four philosophical methodological choices are particularly crucial. These include specific tactical choices about matters of research practice, and overarching challenges about how population health science charts a course within the existing scientific and sociopolitical landscape.

The four challenges featured in the chapter are: (1) how to equitably choose boundaries for the population one researches given populations' heterogeneity; (2) how to balance programs aimed at high-risk populations with programs aimed at the wider population; (3) how to reconcile tensions between programs that treat population health improvement as the ultimate goal vs. programs that treat a broad model of population health concern as a means of fixing the inefficient healthcare system; (4) how to reconcile the desire for "evidence-based" controlled experiments with the difficulty of gathering such evidence about the social determinants of health. I propose guidelines for equitably managing the challenges arising in (1) and (2). I also show that (3) and (4) are rooted in the complex relationship between the various movements and frameworks that have sprung up in recent years as reactions against the failures of the biomedical model of healthcare theory and practice. For example, some population health science scholars agree with evidence-based medicine scholars that randomized controlled trials are the soundest evidence of a treatment's efficacy, but such trials typically test traditional biomedical interventions (drugs, devices, and procedures) but have done far less to assess interventions operating at the level of upstream/fundamental causes or social determinants (economic inequality, inadequate public transportation infrastructure, etc.). The chapter's case study illustrates the issues featured in the chapter by examining ongoing research into the health of global migrants and policy responses to this research.

Chapter 7 argues that health equity concepts are built into population health science and urges a reorienting of the debates over what health equity is and should be:

> we cannot substantially improve the health of the population as a whole without addressing health inequities and ... the drivers of health inequities are often the drivers of the health of the population generally.
>
> (Diez Roux 2016: 619)

Population health science is, as a matter of fact, inseparable from concerns with health equity. The interdisciplinary science of population health itself formed around the goal of revising and expanding public health, with improving health equity as one goal of the reform (Kindig 2007). The relationship between science ethics/normativity has long been a topic of debate for philosophers of science in the "science and values" literature (Elliott and Steel 2017), as well the public health ethics literature disputing whether "population health has an intrinsically distributive dimension" and hence a necessary concern for health equity (Reid 2016: 27). In the case of population health science, issues of equity are built into the science at least as much as any other theoretical component is. This chapter and this book do not seek to offer a competitor theory in the existing literature on the nature of health equity. Instead, it proceeds from philosophical examination of population health *science*, to offer some guidance on the relationship between philosophy and population health science, which includes some points about meta-ethics via critique of how equity concepts can and should function within the population health science community.

I argue that philosophy of public/population health must be more cautious about its assumptions regarding the precise definition and/or moral foundation of health equity. Contrary to a widespread presumption among public health ethicists, we do not need to first achieve a community consensus on either of these before doing good work in public/population health science research or interventions. Indeed, in a diverse world, it is both unrealistic and unethical to reject pluralism about the nuances of what health equity is or what its philosophical foundations are. While I place great value on the scholarship debating these matters, it is imperative that we not assume the endpoint of such debates is that one position wins. For example, I am sympathetic with the "capabilities approach" (Venkatapuram 2011), but do not want this view imposed on others who have alternative conceptions of health equity (Galarneau 2016). As a matter of both philosophy of science and meta-ethics, making headway in health equity debates would be well served by reducing the reliance (especially by philosophers) on hypothetical cases and problems, and increasing attention to the plethora of real (and really messy) cases of health inequities. In a related point, I argue for a shift in health equity deliberations: insofar as health governance and health promotion are two sides of the same coin, (Kickbusch and Gleicher 2012: x), health equity is better served by fostering equitable social structures of health governance. One important piece of that process is ensuring that diverse forms of knowledge, especially the oft-undervalued knowledge held by non-scientists, are respected and included in population health science. The chapter is followed by a case study that illustrates the health equity dynamics discussed in the chapter: the field of scientific research on racial and ethnic health disparities.

Chapter 8 offers "humility" as a guiding philosophical concept for the continued development of a fruitful population health science. The final chapter offers humility as the thread that ties together the disparate strands of population health research and practice. I argue population health experts would be wise to recognize that thread, or risk having the field of population health science unravel. The chapter begins with a restatement of the book's orientation, philosophy of population health in the form of philosophy *for* population health. The book aims to contribute to the project of helping population health science to refine and make progress on its disciplinary path—it is already oriented in the right direction.

The chapter argues that three types of humility are essential to a successful and ethically sound population health science. First, epistemic humility is essential, in that population health science requires open-mindedness on matters such as how non-scientist members of a population can have knowledge about that population. Second, the chapter argues for sectoral humility, since population health science (in its efforts to promote health in all corners of social life) requires intersectoral collaboration between government, non-profits, healthcare companies, and more. Third, interdisciplinary humility is essential because population health science is an interdisciplinary field, which not only requires collaboration between multiple disciplines, but also requires that these must be collaborations among equals—for example, epidemiology has no primacy over medical anthropology. The chapter reflects on some of the challenges of educating future experts in population health science.

What are the book's philosophical methods and commitments?

This book is offered in a spirit of humble interdisciplinary collaboration, expounded in Chapter 8. Philosophy's role in this interdisciplinary project is a unique piece of a whole, and my role in philosophy is likewise just a unique and small piece of a whole. Philosophy is not monolithic—it is many different things and accordingly has many different contributions to make to population health science. What this book can and will bring to the table is largely dictated by the combination of my skill set and the scope of this project as a philosophical study of a branch of science that has not received much previous attention. This book appears in a series titled "History and Philosophy of Biology," and likewise my PhD is in History and Philosophy of Science. With that as my background, this book takes on a more wide-ranging set of literatures and methodologies.

Philosophy of science in practice, as promoted and organized by the Society for Philosophy of Science in Practice, brings the methods and literature of philosophy of science to bear on the philosophy of population health insofar as it features the communities, theories and practices of applied health scientists. "Philosophy of science *in practice*" is used to indicate a respect for the messiness that far too many philosophers of science have tried to set aside in their abstract representations of scientific processes. Population health science is driven by practical goals in health promotion, an endeavor quite unlike the mythologized theoretical physicist's search for universal truths about nature.

Philosophy of medicine is methodologically closely related to philosophy of science in practice, but insofar as medicine is more than just applied science, the philosophy of medicine literature and methods brings a unique ingredient to the book. This book is in part a work of philosophy of medicine, and making sense of population health science will require entering into conversation with both classic debates in the area (e.g., the philosophical nature of health and disease), and emerging topics for the field (e.g., philosophy of causation in epidemiology). To repeat the above point, though, population health science is not a subfield of medicine in a disciplinary sense or in an institutional sense of being part of the healthcare sector. So, this book necessarily includes much outside philosophy of medicine.

Public health ethics and health justice overlap with bioethics and with social and political philosophy, the massive distributive justice literature, and of course have a long history of contending with population-level health. This book will engage with all of these, though the goal of this book is not to offer a direct competitor theory of (public) health justice/equity as others have done (Powers and Faden 2006; Daniels 2008; Ruger 2010; Nussbaum 2011; Venkatapuram 2011). This book is foremost concerned with articulating and defending a view of the philosophical foundations of population health *science*, which in turn sheds light on how the global project of promoting health equity can and should be pursued by diverse practitioners (see Chapter 7). A commitment to coupled ethical-epistemic philosophical practice undergirds my approach to philosophy of population health science (Katikireddi and Valles 2015; Tuana 2013). The ethical and evidentiary aspects of population health science dynamically interact with each other. Population health science requires both ethical rigor and epistemic rigor, and these two features cannot be neatly separated.

The history of population health science is a crucial feature of this book for two reasons. First, as a matter of scholarly practice, I concur with Hansen's famous position that philosophical understandings of a science are vacuous without also examining the corresponding history of science (Hanson 1962). Second, in the case of population health science, attending to the history of the field seems to be the best means of getting a handle on what the field's philosophical commitments are and why. This is why Chapter 2 will present a history of population health science.

Related to my endorsement of philosophy of science in practice, I contend that we should turn to day-to-day practitioners and glean from their own experiences what the pressing philosophical questions are and take it seriously when they offer solutions to them. As an ethically and theoretically motivated reform effort, population health science has always been explicitly engaged with a wide range of abstract and applied philosophical questions. What is health (Kindig 2007)? Who ought to control health governance, and how (Kickbusch 2007)? How can we address the inequitable treatment of marginalized populations in a way that re-empowers them (Government of Western Australia Department of Health 2015)? Some scientific communities may be reluctant to reflect on philosophical matters, but this community is not one of them. This book will reflect that a massive amount of effort has already been profitably spent in sorting out the philosophy of population health science. Some excellent work has certainly been done by professional philosophers (e.g., Goldberg 2009), but population health scientists themselves have produced a body of insightful philosophical literature, largely untapped by professional philosophers.

To be clear, one of the most compelling reasons that this book will engage so closely with the philosophical insights of non-philosopher scholars of population health science (people whose occupations, publication venues and/or scholarly communities place them primarily or entirely outside capital-P-Philosophy) is that paying close attention to them serves the *liberatory project* (see, for example, Medina 2013; Kidd et al. 2017). Oppression and injustice are pervasive, and scholars of population health science have shown an admirable commitment to the global project of liberation. Leading figures in their field have argued passionately for LGBTQ rights and the value of thinking intersectionally about the nexus of sexuality–gender–race, etc. (Galea 2018: 145–150); lucidly contextualized appalling racial health inequities inside even larger patterns of dehumanization, and classist and colonialist disempowerment (Kindig 2017); fought to articulate and proposed international policy steps to address systematic neglect of the diverse indigenous peoples of the far north (Young 2013); and so on. As Chapter 2 will explain, an important piece of population health science's history is its rooting in Latin American radical liberation theories (Diez Roux 2016; Krieger 2011: 163–190). Feminist philosophy, racial health equity scholarship, indigenous epistemology, and all sorts of other liberatory literature—some by philosophers and some not—will appear often in the book. Population health science is, and ought to be, oriented toward justice and liberation and so this book happily follows suit.

What this book is not, and what it will not do

Because this book sits at the intersection of so many areas, and takes on a somewhat amorphous interdisciplinary field of science, the book needs to set a realistic scope. It cannot, and will not attempt to, address every important subfield, topic, dispute, text, argument, etc. related to this sprawling topic. In fact, this is an opportune moment to remind readers that population health science is unique and deserving of intensive philosophical attention in large part *because* it aims to think far more broadly than even the already-broad field of public health. This is not an excuse for any problematic oversights or absences in the upcoming chapters, but it is a reason why the book will necessarily leave many open avenues untraveled. Moreover, when the book does pass up would-be subject matter, it should not be interpreted as an indication that I devalue them—or even that I value them less than the subject matter that is included. Rather, the content that is—and isn't—here is based on my judgments of how I can best articulate, argue for, and synthesize, a cogent cohesive set of contributions to scholarship. As the narrative progresses, I will strive to accompany my arguments with corresponding statements of what I am indeed trying to achieve and why I am trying to achieve it.

I will avoid philosophical jargon and population health science jargon as much as possible in this book. I do this for practical and theoretical reasons. Practically, I wish to spark dialogue between philosophers and population health science professionals, a goal that is best served by speaking to both audiences at the same time. Theoretically, jargon manifests a disciplinary exclusivity that contradict the spirit of inclusivity that I and population health science both endorse. Misunderstandings and knowledge disconnects are inevitable to some extent, but insofar as I share population health science's belief that promoting population health is a collaborative endeavor, it requires efforts to make the conversation as inclusive as possible. It is already limiting enough that I am primarily writing this book for a postgraduate audience.

It is worth taking a moment to acknowledge some of the important questions that I have reluctantly chosen to set aside for the purpose of keeping the book focused on answering a limited set of linked questions. For one, I have set aside the book's planned section on the meaning of "population" since it seems that the question, "what is a population in population health science?" is less pressing a question than I originally anticipated. While Millstein makes a strong case for why a single "population" definition would be desirable in evolutionary biology and ecology, it is less clear that population health science needs a similarly unified concept of population (Millstein 2014). As Kindig surmises, based on Young's population health book, virtually any grouping of people can qualify as a population: geographic region, a nation, global members of a religion, etc. (Kindig 2007). Krieger shows that there are indeed interesting philosophical questions at stake in how and why one uses different population concepts (Krieger 2012; see also the discussion of population lumping vs. splitting in Chapter 6), but I largely leave this question aside in the book.

Future work is needed to further explore the intersections of philosophy of population health science and philosophy of environmental science. Important work has already been done on issues such as philosophy of environmental health (Resnik 2012; Elliott 2011), despite a historical divergence between the literatures of medical bioethics and literatures on the ethics of non-human biological subjects such as non-human animal welfare (Thompson 2015). Yet, issues such as climate change (Chapter 4's case study) create a pressing need for investigations of how population health science and environmental science's respective philosophical issues interrelate (MacPherson 2013; Valles 2015; Dwyer 2009). There will be frequent discussion of environment broadly (safe neighborhoods, etc.), but the environmental philosophy literature will only make limited appearances.

There is also much future work to do on the question of how population health science's discipline formation process meshes with existing philosophy of science theories for how scientific disciplines evolve. Thomas Kuhn's famous "paradigm shift" language (Kuhn 1962) has been used by both supporters (Peterson et al. 2016) and critics (Poland et al. 1998) to describe population health as a genuine scientific revolution, a discontinuous change from older models of public health. Is this an accurate account of what population health science is, or is the field better viewed through the lens of "research program" (better illuminating the continuities with other past and current scientific endeavors; Lakatos 1968) or perhaps "scientific repertoire" (better illuminating the institutional and collaborative influences of the field; Ankeny and Leonelli 2016). Like Miriam Solomon's (2015) and Jeremy Howick's (2011) texts on philosophy of evidence-based medicine, I choose to refrain from devoting the enormous amount of space required to adequately explore if/how this new field technically qualifies as "revolutionary." In a related matter, this book will engage with evidence-based medicine in Chapters 6 and 8, but there is much more work to be done exploring these two parallel efforts to reform health research and practice, all the more so because both emerged in the 1990s out of frustrations with the health science status quo (Evidence-Based Medicine Working Group 1992; Evans et al. 1994).

Onward

Something big has been happening in the world of public health science: an effort to revise, reform, reorient, or arguably even to revolutionize how we think about and practice health promotion for groups of people. I use the term "population health science"; others use "the population health approach" (Arah 2009); "public health 3.0" (DeSalvo et al. 2016); or just what some consider good contemporary public health (Rudolph et al. 2013). Like Diez Roux, I am more concerned about the content of the ideas than the terminology—"the more synonyms we have, the better" (Diez Roux 2016: 620)!

The task ahead is to stitch together fragmentary pieces of insights from many scholars, assembling a cohesive philosophy of population health science. The first step in this process is to turn to the history of population health science.

Works cited

Anderson, G. M., Bronskill, S. E., Mustard, C. A., et al. (2005) Both clinical epidemiology and population health perspectives can define the role of health care in reducing health disparities. *Journal of Clinical Epidemiology* 58, 757–762.

Ankeny, R. A. and Leonelli, S. (2016) Repertoires: A post-Kuhnian perspective on scientific change and collaborative research. *Studies in History and Philosophy of Science Part A* 60, 18–28.

Arah, O. A. (2009) On the relationship between individual and population health. *Medicine, Health Care and Philosophy* 12, 235–244.

Bachrach, C., Robert, S. and Thomas, Y. (2015) *Training in Interdisciplinary Health Science: Current Successes and Future Needs*. Bethesda, MD: National Institutes of Health.

Bell, K. (2017) *Health and Other Unassailable Values: Reconfigurations of Health, Evidence and Ethics*. London: Routledge.

Black, D., Morris, J., Smith, C. and Townsend, P. (1980) Inequalities in Health: Report of a Research Working Group on Inequalities in Health. London: Department of Health and Social Security.

Broadbent, A. (2013) *Philosophy of Epidemiology*. New York: Palgrave Macmillan.

Carel, H. and Cooper, R. (2014) *Health, Illness and Disease: Philosophical Essays*. New York: Routledge.

Carpiano, R. M. and Daley, D. M. (2006) A guide and glossary on postpositivist theory building for population health. *Journal of Epidemiology and Community Health* 60, 564–570.

Commission on Social Determinants of Health. (2008) *Closing the Gap in a Generation: Health Equity Through Action on the Social Determinants of Health*. Geneva: World Health Organization.

Council on Education for Public Health. (2016) Accreditation Criteria: Schools of Public Health & Public Health Programs. Silver Spring, MD: Council on Education for Public Health.

Daniels, N. (2008) *Just Health: Meeting Health Needs Fairly*. New York: Cambridge University Press.

DeSalvo, K. B., O'Carroll, P. W., Koo, D., et al. (2016) Public health 3.0: Time for an upgrade. *American Journal of Public Health* 106, 621–622.

Diez Roux, A. V. (2016) On the distinction—or lack of distinction—between population health and public health. *American Journal of Public Health* 106, 619–620.

Dotson, K. (2015) Philosophy from the Position of Service. In: Krishnamurthy, M. (ed.) *Philosopher*, [blog] edited by Krishnamurthy. https://politicalphilosopher.net/2015/01/09/featured-philosopher-kristie-dotson/.

Dwyer, J. (2009) How to connect bioethics and environmental ethics: Health, sustainability, and justice. *Bioethics* 23, 497–502.

Elliott, K. (2011) *Is a Little Pollution Good for You? Incorporating Societal Values in Environmental Research.* New York: Oxford University Press.

Elliott, K. C. and Steel, D. (2017) *Current Controversies in Values and Science.* London: Routledge.

Evans, R. G., Barer, M. L. and Marmor, T. R. (1994) *Why Are Some People Healthy and Others Not? The Determinants of Health of Populations.* New York: Aldine De Gruyter.

Evidence-Based Medicine Working Group. (1992) Evidence-based medicine: A new approach to teaching the practice of medicine. *Journal of the American Medical Association* 268, 2420–2425.

Fielding, J. E., Kumanyika, S. and Manderscheid, R. W. (2013) A perspective on the development of the Healthy People 2020 framework for improving US population health. *Public Health Reviews* 35, 1–24.

Frank, J. W. (1995) Why "Population Health"? *Canadian Journal of Public Health* 86, 162–164.

Galarneau, C. (2016) *Communities of Health Care Justice.* New Brunswick, NJ: Rutgers University Press.

Galea, S. (2017) Invited commentary: Continuing to loosen the constraints on epidemiology in an age of change—a comment on McMichael's "prisoners of the proximate." *American Journal of Epidemiology* 185, 1217–1219.

Galea, S. (2018) *Healthier: Fifty Thoughts on the Foundations of Population Health.* New York: Oxford University Press.

Goldacre, B. (2012) *Bad Pharma: How Medicine is Broken, and How We Can Fix It.* New York: Faber and Faber, Inc.

Goldberg, D. S. (2009) In support of a broad model of public health: Disparities, social epidemiology and public health causation. *Public Health Ethics* 2, 70–83.

Goldberg, D. S. (2012) Against the very idea of the politicization of public health policy. *American Journal of Public Health* 102, 44–49.

González-Moreno, M., Saborido, C. and Teira, D. (2015) Disease-mongering through clinical trials. *Studies in History and Philosophy of Biological and Biomedical Sciences* 51, 11–18.

Government of Western Australia Department of Health. (2015) WA Aboriginal Health and Wellbeing Framework 2015–2030. http://ww2.health.wa.gov.au/Improving-WA-Health/About-Aboriginal-Health/WA-Aboriginal-Health-and-Wellbeing-Framework-2015-2030: Department of Health.

Hanson, N. R. (1962) The irrelevance of history of science to philosophy of science. *Journal of Philosophy* 59, 574–586.

Health Research & Educational Trust. (2015) Approaches to Population Health in 2015: A National Survey of Hospitals. Chicago: Health Research & Educational Trust.

Hennessy, D. A., Flanagan, W. M., Tanuseputro, P., et al. (2015) The Population Health Model (POHEM): An overview of rationale, methods and applications. *Population Health Metrics* 13, 24.

Hertzman, C., Frank, J. and Evans, R. G. (1994) Heterogeneities in Health Status and the Determinants of Population Health. In: Evans, R. G., Barer, M. L. and Marmor, T. R. (eds) *Why Are Some People Healthy and Others Not?* New York: Aldine De Gruyter.

Howick, J. H. (2011) *The Philosophy of Evidence-Based Medicine.* Oxford: John Wiley & Sons.

Isaac, F. and Gorhan, D. (2016) Making the Case for Population Health Management: The Business Value of a Healthy Workforce. In: Nash, D. B., Fabius, R. J., Skoufalos,

A. et al. (eds) *Population Health: Creating a Culture of Wellness.* Second ed. Burlington, MA: Jones & Bartlett Learning.

Jacobson, D. M. and Teutsch, S. (2012) An environmental scan of integrated approaches for defining and measuring total population health by the clinical care system, the government public health system and stakeholder organizations. Washington, DC: National Quality Forum.

Katikireddi, S. V. and Valles, S. A. (2015) Coupled ethical-epistemic analysis of public health research and practice: Categorizing variables to improve population health and equity. *American Journal of Public Health* 105, e36–e42.

Keyes, K. M. and Galea, S. (2016a) *Population Health Science.* New York: Oxford University Press.

Keyes, K. M. and Galea, S. (2016b) Setting the agenda for a new discipline: Population health science. *American Journal of Public Health* 106, 633–634.

Kickbusch, I. (2003) The contribution of the World Health Organization to a new public health and health promotion. *American Journal of Public Health* 93, 383–388.

Kickbusch, I. (2007) Health governance: The health society. In McQueen, D. V. and Kickbusch, I. (eds) *Health and Modernity.* New York: Springer, 144–161.

Kickbusch, I. and Gleicher, D. (2012) *Governance for Health in the 21st Century.* Copenhagen: World Health Organization Regional Office for Europe.

Kidd, I. J., Medina, J. and Pohlhaus, G. J. (2017) *The Routledge Handbook of Epistemic Injustice.* New York: Routledge.

Kindig, D. (2017) Population health equity: Rate and burden, race and class. *Journal of the American Medical Association* 317, 467–468.

Kindig, D. and Stoddart, G. (2003) What is population health? *American Journal of Public Health* 93, 380–383.

Kindig, D. A. (2007) Understanding population health terminology. *Milbank Quarterly* 85, 139–161.

Krieger, N. (2011) *Epidemiology and the People's Health: Theory and Context.* New York: Oxford University Press.

Krieger, N. (2012) Who and what is a "population"? Historical debates, current controversies, and implications for understanding "population health" and rectifying health inequities. *Milbank Quarterly* 90, 634–681.

Krogsbøll, L. T., Jørgensen, K. J., Grønhøj Larsen, C. and Gøtzsche, P. C. (2012) General health checks in adults for reducing morbidity and mortality from disease. *British Medical Journal* 345, e7191.

Kuhn, T. S. (1962) *The Structure of Scientific Revolutions.* Chicago, IL: University of Chicago Press.

Lakatos, I. (1968) Criticism and the methodology of scientific research programmes. *Proceedings of the Aristotelian society* 69, 149–186.

Lalonde, M. (1974) *A New Perspective on the Health of Canadians.* Ottawa, Canada: Health and Welfare Canada.

Largent, M. A. (2012) *Vaccine: The Debate in Modern America.* Baltimore, MD: Johns Hopkins University Press.

Link, B. G. and Phelan, J. (1995) Social conditions as fundamental causes of disease. *Journal of health and social behavior* 35, 80–94.

MacPherson, C. C. (2013) Climate change is a bioethics problem. *Bioethics* 27, 305–308.

Marmot, M. (2004) *The Status Syndrome: How Social Standing Affects Our Health and Longevity.* New York: Henry Holt and Company.

Marmot, M. G., Shipley, M. J. and Rose, G. (1984) Inequalities in death—specific explanations of a general pattern? *The Lancet* 323, 1003–1006.

McDowell, I., Spasoff, R. A. and Kristjansson, B. (2004) On the classification of population health measurements. *American Journal of Public Health* 94, 388–393.

McQueen, D. V., Wismar, M., Lin, V., et al. (2012) *Intersectoral Governance for Health in All Policies: Structures, Actions and Experiences.* Copenhagen: WHO Regional Office for Europe.

Medina, J. (2013) *The Epistemology of Resistance: Gender and Racial oppression, Epistemic Injustice, and the Social Imagination.* New York: Oxford University Press.

Metzl, J. and Kirkland, A. (2010) *Against Health: How Health Became the New Morality.* New York: New York University Press.

Millstein, R. L. (2014) How the concept of population resolves concepts of environment. *Philosophy of Science* 81, 741–755.

Mir, G., Salway, S., Kai, J., et al. (2013) Principles for research on ethnicity and health: The Leeds Consensus Statement. *The European Journal of Public Health* 23, 504–510.

Murray, C. J. L., Salomon, J. A., Mathers, C. D. and Lopez, A. D. (2002) *Summary Measures of Population Health: Concepts, Ethics, Measurement and Applications.* Geneva: World Health Organization.

Nash, D. B., Fabius, R. J., Skoufalos, A., et al. (2016) *Population Health: Creating a Culture of Wellness.* Second ed. Burlington, MA: Jones & Bartlett Learning.

Nussbaum, M. C. (2011) *Creating Capabilities: The Human Development Approach.* Cambridge: Belknap Press.

Petersen, A. and Lupton, D. (1996) *The New Public Health: Discourses, Knowledges, Strategies.* London: Sage Publications.

Peterson, T. A., Bernstein, S. J. and Spahlinger, D. A. (2016) Population health: A new paradigm for medicine. *The American Journal of the Medical Sciences* 351, 26–32.

Poland, B., Coburn, D., Robertson, A. and Eakin, J. (1998) Wealth, equity and health care: A critique of a "population health" perspective on the determinants of health. *Social Science & Medicine* 46, 785–798.

Powers, M. and Faden, R. R. (2006) *Social Justice: The Moral Foundations of Public Health and Health Policy.* New York: Oxford University Press.

Reid, L. (2016) Does population health have an intrinsically distributional dimension? *Public Health Ethics* 9, 24–36.

Renaud, M. (1994) The Future: Hygeia vs. Panakeia. In: Evans, R. G., Barer, M. L. and Marmor, T. R. (eds) *Why Are Some People Healthy and Others Not?* New York: Aldine De Gruyter.

Resnik, D. B. (2012) *Environmental Health Ethics.* Cambridge: Cambridge University Press.

Rose, G. (1992) *The Strategy of Preventive Medicine.* New York: Oxford University Press.

Rothstein, M. A. (2002) Rethinking the meaning of public health. *The Journal of Law, Medicine & Ethics* 30, 144–149.

Rothstein, M. A. (2009) The limits of public health: A response. *Public Health Ethics* 2, 84–88.

Rudolph, L., Caplan, J., Ben-Moshe, K. and Dillon, L. (2013) *Health in All Policies: A Guide for State and Local Governments.* Washington, DC: American Public Health Association and Public Health Institute.

Ruger, J. P. (2010) *Health and Social Justice.* Oxford: Oxford University Press.

Ruse, M. (2008) Handmaiden to science? *American Scientist* 96, 340–342.

Solomon, M. (2015) *Making Medical Knowledge*. New York: Oxford University Press.

Stoto, M. A. (2013) *Population Health in the Affordable Care Act Era*. Washington, DC: AcademyHealth.

Thompson, P. B. (2015) From synthetic bioethics to One Bioethics: A reply to critics. *Ethics, Policy & Environment* 18, 215–224.

Tricco, A. C., Runnels, V., Sampson, M. and Bouchard, L. (2008) Shifts in the use of population health, health promotion, and public health: A bibliometric analysis. *Canadian Journal of Public Health* 99, 466–471.

Tuana, N. (2013) Embedding philosophers in the practices of science: Bringing humanities to the sciences. *Synthese* 190, 1955–1973.

Valles, S. A. (2012a) Evolutionary medicine at twenty: Rethinking adaptationism and disease. *Biology and Philosophy* 27, 241–261.

Valles, S. A. (2012b) Should direct to consumer personalized genomic medicine remain unregulated? A rebuttal of the defenses. *Perspectives in Biology and Medicine* 55, 250–265.

Valles, S. A. (2015) Bioethics and the framing of climate change's health risks. *Bioethics* 29, 334–341.

Venkatapuram, S. (2011) *Health Justice: An Argument from the Capabilities Approach*. Malden, MA: Polity Press.

Welch, H. G., Schwartz, L. and Woloshin, S. (2011) *Overdiagnosed: Making People Sick in the Pursuit of Health*. Boston, MA: Beacon Press.

Woolf, S. H. and Aron, L. (2013) *US Health in International Perspective: Shorter Lives, Poorer Health*. Washington, DC: National Academies Press.

World Health Organization. (1946) Official Records of the World Health Organization. *International Health Conference*. New York: United Nations.

World Health Organization. (1986) *Ottawa Charter for Health Promotion*. Ottawa, ON: World Health Organization.

World Health Organization. (2011) *Rio Political Declaration on Social Determinants of Health*. Rio de Janeiro: World Health Organization.

World Health Organization. (2014) *Twelfth General Programme of Work 2014–2019: Not Merely the Absence of Disease*. Geneva: World Health Organization.

Xu, J., Murphy, S. L., Kochanek, K. D. and Arias, E. (2016) Mortality in the United States, 2015. *NCHS data brief*, 1–8.

Young, T. K. (1998) *Population Health: Concepts and Methods*. Oxford: Oxford University Press.

Young, T. K. (2005) *Population Health: Concepts and Methods*. New York: Oxford University Press.

Young, T. K. (2013) North-North and North-South Health Disparities. In: Carlson, N., Steinhauer, K. and Goyette, L. (eds) *Disinherited Generations: Our Struggle to Reclaim Treaty Rights for First Nations Women and their Descendants*. Edmonton, Alberta: University of Alberta Press, 211–227.

Part I

What should health mean in population health science?

2 A brief history of the social concept of health and its role in population health science

Introduction

A population health perspective is fundamentally concerned with the social structural nature of health influences, and, although it is embodied in the health outcomes experienced by specific individuals, the domains of influence that shape health experiences transcend the characteristics or circumstances of any one individual (Dunn and Hayes 1999: S7).

The growth of population health science is rooted in a gradual recognition that health is a more social thing than previously acknowledged, in four different senses: metaphysically, empirically, ethically, and methodologically. Population health science emerged from the scientific milieu of mid-late twentieth-century public health and biomedicine, reacting against the status quo that failed to adequately recognize the nature and implications of health as a social phenomenon. This chapter presents the theoretical recognition of those four senses of social health as four stages in the history of population health science's development.

The World Health Organization was founded shortly after the end of World War Two, writing a metaphysically social concept of health into its constitution: "health is a state of complete physical, mental and social well-being and not merely the absence of disease or infirmity" (World Health Organization 1946: 100). But WHO's *metaphysically social* concept of health was quickly suppressed by Cold War-era politics (a combination of fear of socialism and exaltation of technological solutions) (Irwin and Scali 2007). By the 1970s and 1980s, a critical mass of shocking new empirical data had affirmed that health is *empirically social*—the causes and effects of health and disease are fully intertwined in the social fabric of each population (Black et al. 1980). This launched the ongoing efforts to understand the "social determinants of health" (Committee on Educating Health Professionals to Address the Social Determinants of Health 2016). Meanwhile, this new empirical literature buttressed a tradition of recognizing health as *ethically* inseparable from social empowerment. Promoting a population's health is inseparable from promoting social justice within and between populations. The tradition is rooted in nineteenth-century radical social reform, and was advanced in the twentieth century by Latin America's Social Medicine scholars, before finally being recognized in WHO's landmark Ottawa

Charter, which affirmed that promoting a population's health is part and parcel of the social empowerment of that population (World Health Organization 1986). All of those lessons combine to leave the population health science of the late 2010s with an ongoing project: working to refine its theories and practices to make them sufficiently *methodologically* engage with health as a social phenomenon. The most prominent manifestation of this project is the spread of community-based participatory research and related methods, which reconceptualize research subjects as respected research partners, and bearers of practically essential knowledge (Potvin 2007; Wallerstein and Duran 2010).

The biomedical model and the Biostatistical Theory of health

The health science status quo of the mid-late twentieth century is rooted in the biomedical model. Nancy Krieger, a leading population health scholar and developer of the ecosocial model, one of many alternatives to the biomedical model, defines the biomedical model as these three components:

1 "the domain of disease and its causes is restricted to solely biological, chemical, and physical phenomena" (Krieger 2011: 130);
2 "an emphasis on laboratory research and technology," as well as a corresponding disregard for research questions not amenable to experiments via "randomized controlled trials" or observation of "natural experiments" (Krieger 2011: 130);
3 "'reductionism,' a philosophical and methodological stance," according to which, "phenomena are best explained by the properties of their parts" (Krieger 2011: 130).

In the philosophy of medicine literature, Christopher Boorse created a still-influential definition of health that serves as a more formal expression of the health concept operating within the biomedical model (Boorse 1977; Boorse 1975), the Biostatistical Theory of health.

> Health in a member of the reference class is normal functional ability: the readiness of each internal part to perform all its normal functions on typical occasions with at least typical efficiency.
>
> (Boorse 2014: 684)

This view does not reject the notion of health affecting or being affected by social life. It also acknowledges that our social experiences and ethical/evaluative reactions to health and disease are important in medical practice (Boorse 2014). But, this view seats health in objective facts about the workings of components of individual pieces of individual human bodies.

Among many other critiques, Krueger shows Boorse is misguided in building up a person-level concept of health/disease as the net effect of cells/tissues/organs functioning or malfunctioning according to their evolutionary purposes—a pathologist's conception of disease scaled up to the level of the complete person (Krueger 2015). At a given point in time, we are diseased in some respect when a part of our biological machinery malfunctions, or healthy if we lack any such malfunctioning parts. Such a biomedical understanding of health served to prop up the international effort to promote health by prioritizing the development and distribution of drugs and devices that "fix" any "broken" tissues, biochemical pathways, etc. A more socially grounded metaphysics of health remained the official position of the World Health Organization throughout the second half of the twentieth century, the era of peak biomedical model dominance, but WHO endorsement couldn't stand up to more powerful historical influences. A recent *Lancet* series surveying the impediments and solutions to giving the "right care" to patients, singles out "the dominance of the biomedical model" as one important obstacle. It has built up public "prestige" based on its successes and its negative effects overlooked, effects that include, "neglect of patients' cognitive and emotional needs, preferences, underuse of counselling and behavioural therapies, and neglect of social and public health strategies for disease prevention" (Saini et al. 2017: 182). The authors conclude that addressing the full set of "drivers of poor medical care" includes: "re-addressing imbalances of knowledge and power, not only within the clinician-patient relationship but also within delivery systems, and more broadly in society" (Saini et al. 2017: 186). Health science has invested much faith in the biomedical model; now we need to reevaluate by thinking about power and social relations.

Population health as (metaphysically) social health

According to the World Health Organization's Constitution: "Health is a state of complete physical, mental and social well-being and not merely the absence of disease or infirmity" (World Health Organization 1946: 100). This is a bold assertion about the metaphysics of health. It offers a clear alternative to the biomedical model of health. But countervailing historical forces suppressed its influence for decades.

WHO had an inconsistent history of acting in accordance with its own metaphysical concept of health (Irwin and Scali 2007, 2010). Writing for a WHO discussion forum, Irwin and Scali chastise WHO for losing sight of its founding definition of health (Irwin and Scali 2010). They explain that WHO's nearly immediate post-founding pivot to a technology-centered biomedical model of health is largely attributable to a combination of two factors. First, the fashionable 1950s technocratic ideology prioritized biomedical efforts such as vaccine development. Second, the US's growing political and financial power over WHO coincided with its growth as a Cold War superpower, afraid that emphasizing health's collective and social features would cede ground to its communist and socialist foes (Irwin and Scali 2007). The US was not wrong to see a connection between social conceptions of health and political socialism. As elaborated below, social conceptions of health have their roots in revolutionary communist and socialist social justice movements. And, as also elaborated below, the US's dismal public health record is the starkest illustration of the biomedical model's faults.

WHO's decision to advance such an obviously disputable metaphysical position at its precarious founding moment in the aftermath of World War Two still made strategic sense in part because that holistic definition freed its hands to pursue all manner of health promotion activity without being held back by too narrow a mandate. If WHO had been chartered to only prevent disease, to constrain its efforts to communicable diseases, or to only work towards certain benchmarks (life expectancy, infant mortality, etc.) then it could easily have been left in situations where it sought to promote health in ways it was not explicitly authorized to do. In addition to the pragmatic benefits of a broad mandate, WHO's founding commitment to an intrinsically social concept of health is a natural extension of the mission of the United Nations, its parent organization. WHO's definition of health appeared in the preamble to the WHO Constitution alongside a series of similarly bold philosophical assertions, all of which mesh well with the ambitious global peace and justice mission of the UN. According to the WHO Constitution's preamble: health is a prerequisite for "peace and security" (echoing the UN charter drafted the previous year); it advocates for interpersonal and international cooperation (much like the UN); and it complements the UN charter's assertions about human rights, in part by tracing routes for achieving those human rights (including "the ability to live harmoniously in a changing total environment") (World Health Organization 1946: 100). The breadth of the WHO concept of health as social well-being is partly an outgrowth of the breadth of the UN peace and justice mandate.

The metaphysical conception of health as social was bolstered by the historical growth of life course theory in biomedical and social sciences, including epidemiology. And, in turn, life course theory will be central to the concept of health I propose in Chapter 3. Life course theory sees individuals and populations as entities that develop dynamically over time and interactively with their environments. Human lives are not lived in biologically isolated bodies, nor do lives exist as a series of separable slices in time. Human lives are social, lived in dynamic interactions with the humans and non-humans in our environments, and each moment in a life is situated in a life trajectory, shaped by the life history that preceded it and facing its future with the direction set by that history. "Life course" theory and "population health" follow remarkably close patterns of disciplinary developments—both had existed as sporadically used terms and had theoretical antecedents, but each coalesced in the mid-1990s. The roots of life course theory reach as deep as the early twentieth century, drawing on developments in demography, family studies and longitudinal study designs, arguing that human lives should be understood as developing and evolving over time within a social context (Elder et al. 2003). Shanahan et al. point to a 1990 "tipping point," after which life course theory publications began growing exponentially in sociology, psychology, and "biomedical/epidemiology" (Shanahan et al. 2016), much as "population health" grew exponentially starting in the 1990s (Figure 1.1). Today, life course theory is so fundamental to population health theory that Keyes and Galea list it as one of their ten "foundational principles of population health science": "The causes of population health are multi-level, accumulate throughout the life course, and are embedded in dynamic interpersonal relationships" (Keyes and Galea 2016: xiii). The Whitehall Study, discussed in the next section, foreshadowed the eventual synthesizing of life course epidemiology with social determinants theory by unexpectedly finding that taller participants had lower mortality than their shorter peers, suggesting health experiences before adulthood have lifelong effects (Marmot et al. 1984). But, historically, I wish to stress that the metaphysical view of health as a social phenomenon *preceded* the accumulation of some of the most compelling empirical data that shows the multitude of causal pathways by which human health is embedded in sociality.

Health is (empirically) social

As an empirical matter of which causes serve as the main drivers of health, health is social. The growth of attention to "population health" since the 1990s is, first and foremost, a process of responding to new empirical findings. The empirical linchpin in establishing health as inherently and irreducibly social was the development of "social determinants of health" data and theory. Before this literature was firmly established it was possible to credibly claim that the obvious differences in health status between different populations (e.g., infectious disease among the poor) could be explained away as superficial features distracting from the real causes and relationships. Indeed, opponents of social determinants of health scholarship ordered explanations that tried to reduce social inequalities down to a series of factors acting at the individual level. This reductionist backlash is best illustrated in the reception of the UK's landmark Black Report.

James House frames the Black Report as a turning point for the biomedical model (House 2015). The report on population inequalities in the country's universal health insurance program—named for lead author Sir Douglas Black—found that universal healthcare had not eliminated class disparities in health; it may have even widened some disparities (House 2015: 57). This was a remarkable finding, since the establishment of a universal socialized medical system, the National Health Service, would have been expected under a biomedical model to make massive headway in evening out the health experiences of the rich and the poor. If healthcare for individual patients is what drives health then a single universal system giving virtually free treatment to all should have made massive progress in raising up the impoverished and making their health converge with the health of the wealthy. It didn't. This presented a conundrum. That is, if the availability of individual healthcare, under the individualistic and pathology-centered biomedical model of health, did not yield health for all recipients thereof, then some other powerful factor(s) must be at play. The report surmised that healthcare, even the country's universal and largely cost-free system, played a smaller role in population health disparities than the role played by everyday social life:

Whilst the healthcare services can play, and do play, a significant part in reducing inequalities in health, yet measures to reduce differences in material standards of living as experienced at work, in the home and in everyday social and community life are of even greater importance.

(Black et al. 1980)

This diminishment of the power of medicine and elevation of the power of social life was radical.

The authors of the Black Report reviewed candidate explanations for what could be causing the disparities, and ultimately favored explanations attributing the inequalities to the presence of social deprivations rather than the other proposed explanations: statistical artifact, individual misbehavior, or backwards causation (low social class is a consequence of bad individual-level health, rather than the other way around) (Black et al. 1980; Yadavendu 2014: 149–153). In other words, in their favored explanation, population health disparities were not reducible to non-social factors. The observed vast disparities were not explainable as a statistical artifact signifying nothing; nor as the sum of independent bad behaviors by individuals; nor were they explainable by the hypothesis that ill health causes poverty (the converse of the position argued by social determinants of health theorists). Empirical data had shown that health is determined, to an astounding degree, by social causes. This conclusion flew in the face of conservative ideology that views individuals as makers of their own destinies, and the sick as victims of some combination of bad personal choices, bad individual luck, and inborn weakness. This may seem to be reading too much into the significance of the report, but the incoming Thatcher government's fear of the report is evidence of its significance.

The Black Report was commissioned during the liberal government of James Callaghan but completed after the ascendance of the conservative Thatcher government. The report on persistent economic and health inequality was, of course, unappealing to individualistic and economic laissez-faire conservative ideology. So, the government suppressed the report, releasing only 260 copies—unbound copies no less—quietly released over a holiday weekend (Berridge 2002). This same pattern was repeated with the release of Margaret Whitehead's 1987 *Health Divide* report showing growing economic inequality in the 1980s, leading to yet another attempt to muffle announcements of the data, which in turn led to media stories alleging a cover-up (Marmot 2004: 239–240). This empirical data is politically dangerous.

Yadavendu argues that the Black Report and the related literature were groundbreaking, more because of their explanations of health disparities than their confirmation that the disparities exist in the first place (Yadavendu 2014). I agree, but it was also important that the report offered such a thorough and quantitative survey of the empirical data on health disparities between social groups. Other studies followed suit. In the mid-1980s, the US government's Heckler Report examined racial disparities in US health (Secretary's Task Force on Black and Minority Health 1985). In the UK, in the wake of the 1980 Black

Report, Michael Marmot's Whitehall Study soon began releasing its most striking results showing the power of socioeconomic status as a social determinant of health.

The Whitehall Study had the epistemic/evidentiary benefit of controlling many of the variables that had left the Black Report's authors hesitant to render firm conclusions about the causal factors behind health disparities in the UK (Black et al. 1980). Are disparities due to geography, type of occupation, or any factors related to these? The Whitehall Study controlled for these by examining only men (and yes, it was unfortunately only men) within a single occupational hierarchy: "office-based civil servants in London" (Marmot et al. 1984: 1003). Its most important innovation was showing that health–wealth relationship affects all social classes, not just the very poor (Marmot et al. 1984). Moreover, the Whitehall data echoed the Black Report's finding that universal healthcare did not eliminate health disparities; Marmot et al.'s data showed "access to or quality of medical care" was not a major contributor to the disparity between the social classes' differential health outcomes (Marmot et al. 1984: 1006).

Marmot recounts that a shocking outcome of the Whitehall data was the empirical finding that class and health connections travel all the way up the socioeconomic ladder (Marmot 2004). The connection between health and wealth is more than just a function of the travails of poverty. For example, recent data in the US shows the gradient line travels smoothly upward from the 1st income percentile through the 99th (Chetty et al. 2016). As verified in subsequent studies in populations across the globe, we are *all* sitting somewhere on a population health–wealth gradient—the poorest die young, the richest have long lives, and all those between sit on a smooth gradient between the extremes. None are exempted from the social nature of health—rich and poor alike have individual health constantly and inescapably shaped by social factors. We are all sitting on the same hill, some nearer to the top, and some on the steeper slope near the bottom, but we are all standing on tilted ground, looking up at the wealthier/healthier and down at the poorer/less healthy.

Marmot had worked with epidemiologist Geoffrey Rose on the Whitehall Study, and both went on to be leaders in making the empirical case for health as an empirically social phenomenon. Rose had set up the Whitehall Study with influential epidemiologist Donald Reid (Marmot and Brunner 2005). However, Reid and Rose both died relatively young, in their 60s; Reid died of a heart attack in 1977, before the most famous Whitehall findings emerged, and Rose died of cancer in 1993, shortly after completing his book, *The Strategy of Preventive Medicine* (Rose 1992). Highlighted in Chapter 5, Rose's work distinguished between the "causes of cases" of disease (e.g., HIV infection causes a patient to have AIDS) from "causes of incidence" that drive disparities between populations (e.g., populations' AIDS rates vary due to their access to factors such as condoms and sterile paraphernalia for injection drug use). And, highlighted in Chapter 6, Rose's work also articulated his famous "population approach" to health promotion, favoring interventions designed to positively impact all of a society's members. The early deaths of Rose and Reid left

Marmot as the chief voice of the Whitehall study, the leader of the Whitehall II follow-up study, and the leading personage in the ever-expanding literature on the social determinants of health. Meanwhile, Rose is hailed by Keyes and Galea as the founder of population health science.

Much like Gregor Mendel's data on pea plant genetics was not immediately extrapolated to inheritance in other species (Smocovitis 1996), there was also reasonable doubt that the Whitehall data on the health–wealth gradient might be confined to the UK and perhaps some other countries with strong class systems (Marmot 2004: 3). Instead, the health–wealth gradient and social determinants of health have been confined and reconfirmed, with local variations on the theme, again and again (Marmot 2004; Commission on Social Determinants of Health 2008). Globally, health is empirically social.

Promoting health is ethically tied to social empowerment

As Galea puts it, "… social justice is so central to public health that it becomes, paradoxically, easy to overlook" (Galea 2018: 12). But understandings of social justice are diverse and historical trends therein have shifted them over time. Written in the historical midst of a wave of empirical data on health's empirical grounding as a social phenomenon, the 1986 Ottawa Charter for Health Promotion is a landmark WHO document that laid the groundwork for contemporary population health science by crystallizing the ethical goals for health promotion efforts. The most crucial element was setting empowerment as a goal of health promotion efforts: "health promotion is the process of enabling people to increase control over, and to improve, their health"; accordingly, "at the heart of this process is the empowerment of communities, their ownership and control of their own endeavours and destinies" (World Health Organization 1986). In the process, the Ottawa Charter set the stage for several key features of contemporary population health science: its advancing of multi-sectoral action on health, for example, the "health in all policies model," (featured in Chapter 4), and respect for diverse forms of expertise, including the expertise laypeople have in their own community affairs (featured in Chapters 3, 7, and 8). It sought "to reorient health services and their resources towards the promotion of health; and to share power with other sectors, other disciplines and most importantly with people themselves" (World Health Organization 1986).

The groundwork for the Ottawa charter was laid by a combination of the 1978 Declaration of Alma-Ata composed at a WHO- and UNICEF-sponsored conference, and the 1981 *Global Strategy for Health for All by the Year 2000*. The Declaration of Alma-Ata, the better known of the two, affirmed that "health for all the people of the world" is a goal that "requires the action of many other social and economic sectors in addition to the health sector" (International Conference on Primary Health Care 1978). "Health for All" became cemented as the (continuing) motto for global health equity efforts after it was reiterated in a 1981 WHO report, *Global Strategy for Health for All by the Year 2000* (World Health Organization 1981). The Ottawa Charter explicitly frames itself as a continuation of Alma-Ata's earlier and less complete articulation of similar themes. Health for All was, of course, not going to be strictly possible (no one expected death and disease to be conquered by the year 2000), but it set an ethical aspiration. That aspiration makes more sense if understood within the context of the WHO definition of health as the positive presence of well-being, not just the absence of disease. Under such a "positive" health concept, there are no strict endpoints for the health of even a single person—perfect or even virtually perfect health cannot exist in anyone, so all health improvement efforts must aspire to move forward, but not to reach an endpoint. Critics object to health improvement goals without endpoints (Daniels 2006), but this does not stop us from working to make health better—for all. Chapter 3 lays out my case for adopting this health concept: *Health is a life course trajectory of complete well-being in social context.*

The importance of the 1986 Ottawa Charter can hardly be overstated. First and foremost, it offered a vision of population health promotion with an ethics of social empowerment at its core, and made social justice inseparable from health promotion (Catford 2011). As summarized by Kickbusch, a scholar of social determinants of health and leader in the writing of the charter, it "involved the citizens and the communities themselves in a participatory process" of creating health (Kickbusch 2007: 156). Moreover, its:

> definition of health promotion first and foremost recognizes people as social actors and agents and has a focus on their empowerment in the sense of life-politics: health promotion is the process to increase control of people over their health.
>
> (Kickbusch 2007: 156)

Historically, the Ottawa Charter was a bold reaffirmation of WHO's purpose in an era of institutional crisis. The late 1980s through early 1990s saw WHO eclipsed by the World Bank, whose "population and health" lending funds alone exceeded the entire WHO budget (Irwin and Scali 2010: 17). But WHO entered the 1990s committed to the direction set in the Ottawa Charter, reaffirming "health equity as primarily related to people's positions within social hierarchies, and thus to gradients of social, economic and political power" (Irwin and Scali 2010: 18). This attention to social factors as social determinants was reinvigorated by the adoption of the UN Millennium Development Goals in 2000, a set of health and social equity goals (e.g., women's empowerment; child mortality reduction), which necessitated collaborative health promotion efforts between multiple sectors of society, not just healthcare (Irwin and Scali 2010). WHO had been moving in this direction—toward a "health in all policies" approach to health promotion since the 1978 Declaration of Alma-Ata had challenged policymakers to look at more than the clinic in their efforts to improve health (International Conference on Primary Health Care 1978; Centers for Disease Control and Prevention 2015).

The ethical legacy of the Ottawa Charter lives on, despite a plethora of subsequent declarations, reports, treaties, and such from WHO and other prominent organizations. Among other indicators, it has been celebrated in commissioned journal issues (Catford 2011) and articles (Potvin and Jones 2011), and cited as the ethical foundation for a recent joint statement led by the European Public Health Association, decrying decades of European underinvestment in public health and the rise of political oppression against migrants, religious minorities and other socially vulnerable populations (McKee et al. 2016).

But the WHO developments did not happen in a vacuum. Scholars from across the globe had been developing ethical stances on the ethics of population health sciences, population health policy and population health promotion. Most notably, Latin America was pushing the ethical agenda forward. In tracing the history of what distinguishes "population health" from "public health," Diez Roux (2016) and Labonté et al. (2005) both trace lines of historical influence from Latin American social medicine's concepts of "saude coletiva ['salud colectiva'; collective health]," developed in the 1970s. Both articles also extend the historical line of influence all the way to Evans and Stoddart's 1990 article (Evans and Stoddart 1990), an article which was republished and synthesized with a collection of work by scholars at the Canadian Institute for Advanced Research, in a 1994 volume, *Why Are Some People Healthy and Others Not?* (Evans et al. 1994). In his role as the foremost advocate for population health thinking in the wider biomedical community, Kindig cites this 1994 volume as the preeminent text on the topic. I agree. As seen in Figure 1.1, from the mid-1990s to 2016, the term "population health" has been making increasing gains in PubMed entries, relative to "public health."

This favoring of an empowerment-centered social ethic for population health co-evolved with the empirical understanding of health as social. As Evans and Stoddart observed in their pivotal 1990 article, an empowered sense of personal efficacy—the trait of confidence in one's ability to carry out life plans—is empirically linked to socioeconomic status and the phenomena of health-related life choices (1990: 1357):

> The sense of personal efficacy associated with higher social position encourages beliefs both in one's ability to break addictions, and in the positive consequences of doing so. Beliefs in the effectiveness (or lack of it) of one's own actions are both learned, and reinforced by one's social position.
>
> (Evans and Stoddart 1990: 1357)

As an empirical matter, empowerment is necessary for people to carry out healthy life plans. As explored in more recent scholarship, promoting the ethical goal of empowerment has the further benefit of illuminating the complexities of disability and addressing the ethical failures of ableism. Empowering communities and the people within them to take control over their lives allows them to be healthier, even in the presence of many biological disabilities or pathologies. The presence of a "disability" such as deafness does not intrinsically or automatically mean one's health is worse off (Campbell and Stramondo 2017). One reason is that, in many cases, a person with a disease or disability can "adapt" to it, in the sense of not just changing their attitude or expectations, but genuinely changing their health, such as the way that one can adapt to a hand injury by learning to do tasks with the other hand and thus gradually reducing the health harm of having a disabled hand (Salomon and Murray 2002). But adaptations and other factors that facilitate well-being among the disabled are largely controlled at the social level. A supportive and empowering community is conducive to the well-being of all of its members, those with biological pathologies and those without. In ableist non-supportive communities, having a physical disability makes one much more liable to be socially isolated—but it is the isolation, not the physiological pathology, that lowers the well-being (Amundson 2005). Moreover, the problem of isolation is not only something that can be ameliorated at the social level—all members of a community are bene-fitted by making the community less isolating (Amundson 2005).

To summarize: (1) Empowerment is crucial for good health by definition if one adopts the metaphysical position of WHO (again, I will say in Chapter 3 why we should do so); (2) Empowerment was adopted as an ethical goal for health pro-motion partly on its own merits; (3) the case for why empowerment should be ethically central to health promotion is partly related to the solidifying body of empirical data showing that disempowered people make unhealthy life choices (regardless of how one specifies the definition of health). Meanwhile, the Latin American social medicine influence on the ethical commitment to empowerment and a social ethics of health continued to make an impact on WHO and the public health community; and (4) Empowerment makes health more achievable for those who do have disabilities or pathologies, since the harms of such pathol-ogies are, to a large degree, mediated by empowering or disempowering social structures.

Krieger has sought to keep the revolutionary spirit of public health alive, a spirit present since the origins of public health science, which was born in the milieu of mid-nineteenth-century social radicalism and social justice (global popular revolts against oppressive regimes; abolitionism; the birth of com-munism, etc.) (Krieger 2011; Krieger and Birn 1998). After all, Friedrich Engels was a scholar studying the social origins of laborers' health ills in the days before he co-authored the *Communist Manifesto* as an ethical and political solu-tion to the injustices he had seen in his data (Waitzkin 2007). Latin American Social Medicine scholars point to 1848, the pinnacle of this radical era, as the origin of their movement linking social justice and social health (Granda 2008), and Krieger traces the "Spirit of 1848" spirit to today (she leads the Spirit of 1848 caucus of the American Public Health Association), through the intermedi-ary of Latin American Social Medicine, and chastises her colleagues for neglect-ing this tradition (Krieger 2011: 189).

Waitzkin has shown the deep connections between the empirical and the ethical dimensions of social health by examining the roots of social health in Latin American Social Medicine (Waitzkin 2007). As explained in Chapter 1, there is a surprisingly wide gulf between contemporary population health science research and social medicine. Yet, social medicine played a pivotal role in the creation of a global literature on health as a social ethical issue. Perhaps the most fitting, tragically poignant illustration of the power of these collective health ideals is the fate of Salvador Allende, a crucial developer of Latin American social medicine and collective health theory. His foregrounding of anti-imperialism and empowerment through radical social transformation earned the trust of his fellow Chileans, who elected him president. Imperialism fought back, and the socialist president committed suicide during a US-backed coup in 1973.

The influence of Latin America's social medicine tradition lives on in the ongoing refinement of strategies for methodologically contending with health as a social entity. Perhaps the most important influence on contemporary population health science is the influence of that Latin American tradition on the development of new "community-based participatory research" methods, which have drastically shifted the theory and practice of population health research (among many other branches of research). These participatory methods, featured in the next section, were pushed by the Pan American Health Organization, which in turn drew upon support from Latin American social medicine and collective health, including the organization Brazilian Association of Graduates in Collective Health (Granda 2004; Working Group on Healthy Municipalities and Communities 2005). Chapter 5's case study of the AIDS response in Brazil will show another example of the continuing influence of social medicine ideology.

An ethical commitment to health as a social phenomenon leads smoothly into a preference for research methods that reflect this sociality. In fact, the ethical and methodological views of social health travel together with the empirical view of social health. Historian Simon Szreter contextualizes the growth of the "population health approach" within the long history of interplay between public health changes, the study of those changes, and efforts by the powers-that-be to link population health considerations to laissez-faire economics (most recently in the form of neo-liberal economics) (Szreter 2005: 36–42). Szreter's historical narrative of population health points to the World Bank's milestone *Voices of the Poor* report, which endorsed the importance of "empowerment … and relations of mutual respect and support" in health promotion (Szreter 2003: 428; see also Szreter 2005: 39–40); methodologically, it reached these conclusions by systematically collecting testimony from people around the world and actually taking that testimony seriously. Indeed, as Carel and Kidd have argued in the healthcare context, there are grave dangers of committing "epistemic injustice"—the injustice of undermining someone's abilities or credibility as a knower (Fricker 2007)—by sidelining the testimony of those who report suffering; and enormous ethical benefits to correcting that injustice—which partially rests on the unsound empirical assumption that the ill are unreliable reporters of their own experiences and needs—by genuinely listening (Carel and Kidd 2014). Chapter 8 will continue this discussion of epistemic humility, arguing it is essential for the success of population health science.

Methodologies of health research and health promotion must engage with health as a social phenomenon

Moving away from a focus on individual(istic) behavior was central to the development of population health thinking. And the biomedical model of health is the best-established manifestation of a view of health as a collection of physiological functionings or pathologies in individual bodies. Disputes over the biomedical model led to a series of reactions against the model throughout the twentieth century, with population health approaches being one (somewhat heterogeneous) set of reactions. That is, not all who endorse population health-thinking or approaches fully reject the biomedical model, but population health-thinking emerges from the reactions to the biomedical model.

Data undermining the biomedical model is politically dangerous, in just the same way that the 1980 Black Report's data was dangerous for undermining individualistic conservative social welfare policies. Historically, the biomedical model had received a similar challenge in a prominent government report, the 1974 Lalonde Report, a concise text by Marc Lalonde, the Canadian Minister of National Health and Welfare under Pierre Trudeau's liberal government (Lalonde 1974). Also in the mid-1970s, Thomas McKeown became a gadfly to the biomedical model by arguing, on the basis of historical interpretation and empirical data, that medicine and the biomedical model had played far more limited roles in the previous century of health improvements than generally believed (McKeown 1976). Lalonde's and McKeown's work shared the strange distinction of inspiring widely varying conclusions among readers.

The Lalonde report announced that the biomedical model being used at the time was inadequate, and warned that a new, broader, and better-synchronized approach to health promotion was necessary. The report proposed the "Health Field Concept," the mobilization and coordination of all sectors of society affecting health, rather than concentrating health efforts on the healthcare sector. One consequence of that concept was to give an early push for an intersectoral integration of efforts, which later became a central feature of population health science (see Chapter 8), for example, improving nutrition through a combination of school education, general public education, nutritional regulation, etc. in addition to healthcare efforts (Kickbusch 2003). But others saw the Lalonde Report as an articulation of public health failures that required re-doubling efforts to refine and fund the current model of practice, the biomedical model, seeing that "lifestyle" had just as high a billing as "environment" in the report's breakdown of the determinants of health (Irwin and Scali 2007). When combined with the report's advocacy of attending to individual risk factors, the report served as a justification for attempts to endlessly parse risk factors and to victim-blame people for their lifestyle-related ills rather than blaming the societal structures that make healthy individual lifestyles difficult to achieve (Irwin and Scali 2007).

Simon Szreter's 2003 history article, and the related section of his 2005 book, argues that population health approaches (or at least the subset that he investigates) have served to bolster the neo-liberal ideology and laissez-faire economics of US conservatism (Szreter 2003, 2005: 23–42). He points to McKeown's famous macro-analysis of the relative importance of different factors in contributing to the last two centuries' trend of increasing life expectancy (Szreter 2003; McKeown 1976). Even setting aside, for the moment, the continuing debate over the relative contributions of healthcare, genetics, and other factors to overall population health (McGovern et al. 2014). The neo-liberal interpretation of McKeown's work, highlighted in Szreter's history, is only one of the disparate interpretations. On the other end of the spectrum, James begins his book with a quote from McKeown, then proceeds to attack the bio-medical model as both ineffectual and actively harmful, defending McKeown's data showing the importance of public sanitation and other such efforts as evidence that McKeown's data suggests the need for liberal interventionist policies, not laissez-faire neo-liberal capitalism (James 2015: 23). Similarly, public health ethicist Reid has fought back against attempts to use McKeown's data and related literature to argue against attempts to undermine universal healthcare and instead devote the funds to social reforms—a false dichotomy (Reid 2015). Such is the challenge of determining how to proceed methodologically once empirical data suggest healthcare is causally weaker than expected—Chapters 5 and 6 will contend with this in more detail.

The ambiguous lessons of Lalonde's and McKeown's work churned in the background in subsequent years, eventually inspiring Evans and Stoddart to begin working toward a new positive model for health promotion, one more sharply defined than Lalonde's outline (Evans and Stoddart 1990; MacDonald et al. 2013). And, as reported by the editors of the 1994 volume that launched contemporary population health research (in which Evans and Stoddart's article was republished), the combination of work by Marmot, Lalonde, McKeown and some other scholars jointly inspired the creation of the volume that made "population health" a distinct subject of study (Evans et al. 2010).

The new field of population health science took population heterogeneity and distribution of experiences to be central. The newly proposed question was not "why is this population healthy/unhealthy on average?"; the question was, as bluntly put in the title of the 1994 volume, *Why Are Some People Healthy and Others Not?* (Evans et al. 1994). Population variation was suddenly front and center for the new public/population health scholars, and new methods had to be developed to contend with this variation. In the mid-1990s, Link and Phelan developed their Fundamental Cause Theory (which I promote in Chapter 5), having inferred from McKeown's work the importance of social factors such as education and pollution regulations (Link and Phelan 1995; Link and Phelan 2002). Rose—Marmot's erstwhile collaborator and a founding figure of population health theory—went on to develop his own theoretical stance on health promotion, partly reacting against the risk-focused tradition that Lalonde had helped inspire. Rather than medically managing high-risk subpopulations, Rose sought to develop population-wide interventions as a means of helping people from across the diverse varieties of behaviors and social experiences in any large population. He pointed out, "the efforts of individuals are only likely to be effective when they are working with the societal trend" and that "the behavior and health of [society's] individual members are profoundly influenced by its collective characteristics and social norms"; the good news, though, is that these "can be changed either by the behavior of individuals, such as opinion formers and health educators, or by the mass effects of changes in the economy, the environment, or technical developments" (Rose 1992: 62). Individualistic attempts to effect change, one patient at a time, are doomed to failure—changing a population's health requires changing the basic social norms governing every member of that society. "Individual" lifestyle choices are an illusion—those choices are inextricably social and must be addressed with methods that recognize this.

The nature of health as metaphysically social and as ethically inseparable from social empowerment comprise a double challenge to the methods used in population health research. If health is a state of positive holistic well-being, inseparable from societal contexts, are our methods well suited for analyzing such phenomena? If health is ethically inseparable from empowerment, are our methods well suited for promoting such empowering populations? Shortly after the 1986 Ottawa Charter established health as ethically inseparable from social empowerment, WHO went on to advocate for corresponding "participatory research" methodologies (WHO Regional Office for Europe 1988). In fact, participatory research—the genuine and thorough integration of community members into the research aiming to benefit them—should have been sufficiently justified by simply the acknowledgment of health as a metaphysically social entity. If health is holistic social well-being then how could it be rigorously assessed without extensive consultation with those whose holistic well-being is being investigated? By the 1990s, though, it was getting hard to justify the traditional division of knowledge-related labor in research, under which research subjects were treated as data points rather than knowers. Nancy McHugh offers illuminating philosophical case study analyses of what it looks like to do this; unsurprisingly, the details are everything (McHugh 2015). If health is social then community members are experts in their own health contexts and hence have vital information that must be incorporated at every stage of the research process, from choosing which questions merit investigation ("upstream"), through the process of sharing findings and deliberating next steps ("downstream").

The problem of insufficient participatory research was recognized and forcefully challenged in the 1993 Leeds Declaration, an influential document composed during a multidisciplinary workshop that produced a ten-item statement of "New Approaches to Population Health Research and Practice." Among the other items, it decreed:

> Lay people are experts and experts are lay people—lay knowledge about health needs, health services priorities and health outcomes should be central to public health research.
>
> (The Leeds Declaration, in The Lancet Editors 1994)

The statement was favorably received by audiences ranging from the editors of the definitively mainstream *The Lancet* (The Lancet Editors 1994) to the pages of the more radical journal, *Critical Public Health* (Long 1997). As *The Lancet*'s editors explained, many epidemiologists had focused so intently on attempts to investigate *disease*, and uncover the objective universal truths of biology and behavior, that they had neglected the study/promotion of *health* and neglected WHO's 1988 recommendation in support of "participatory research," research capable of reflecting the experiences of the people whom they sought to serve (The Lancet Editors 1994). Chapter 5 will expand on the concern over whether disease or health is the subject of concern for epidemiologists, in its discussion of the medical sociologist Aaron Antonovsky's influential model of salutogenesis, an attempt to reorient health promotion away from disease and toward health (see Mittelmark et al. 2017).

The pursuit of "participation" and "empowerment" are necessary for two distinct reasons, which can actually serve to muddle discussions of their value. Empowering and participatory methods are essential for both proper goals in their own right and they are also instrumental goals that serve other goals. Insofar as health is well-being under the UN model (discussed above, defended in detail in Chapter 3), it is anathema to individual/population health to disempower, and certainly anathema to *social well-being* to exclude people from the social processes and policies in which they have rightful stakes. But the achievement of health promotion goals of all sorts is aided by the incorporation of participatory methods as a means, especially considering that population health interventions of any kind (e.g., exercise programs for children) rely on community commitment to keep running when the grant ends, or the when the policymaker is out of the room. It is foolish to ignore how "power and agency" affect health promotion efforts (Freudenberg and Tsui 2014: 13). For instance, Burke describes the problem of how signed language accommodations are managed in the US, a process in which deaf people submit requests to organizations (e.g., the organizers of a conference), but then the requesters are left out of the process of choosing which interpretive services are offered, and must rely on whichever interpreter shows up at the designated time and place (Burke 2017). This directly undermines the social inclusion goals of disability accommodation laws—the deaf community members are being excluded from the process of how they are nominally being included. And this inclusion also undermines the achievement of even the basic function of reliably matching translation services with the particular needs of each deaf person—without participation, deaf people are often ill-served by interpreters who lack the right skill set for the context (Burke 2017).

Like their peers in other disciplines interested in participatory research, population health science researchers struggle to fully respond to the challenge of reforming research to be thoroughly participatory (Potvin 2007). The central challenge is that participatory research requires both flexibility in one's research questions/hypotheses/methods, and skills that would otherwise be unnecessary (e.g., knowing how to work collaboratively with non-scientists). It is abundantly clear, though, to researchers and even to wealthy funding agencies, that the participatory shift is ethically desirable ("democratizing science") and epistemically desirable ("partnering with community members to best contextualize an intervention for specific settings"), and generally pragmatically desirable ("integrating cultural values and practices to enhance sustainability when grant funding ends") (Wallerstein and Duran 2010: S44). The twenty-first century has seen the fruition of multiple models of community-based participatory research, and all manner of kindred models of scientific research that respects laypeople as legitimate and desirable contributors in the scientific process. Laypeople are more than objects to be prodded and scrutinized in research, or uncritical consumers to be fed scientific knowledge. The payoff of these new participatory methods is that there are ample reasons to believe that they yield robustly superior empirical knowledge. This is the final thread in the network of connections between the interconnected elements of health as social entity: metaphysical, empirical, ethical, and methodological.

Conclusion: moving toward a thoroughly social concept of health

It is not novel to say that individuals' or groups' health is social. Here I have made the stronger claim that health is properly understood as social in four related ways: the metaphysics of health, the empirical data about population health patterns, the ethics of population health and the methods for investigating and promoting people's health. What I have sketched in the preceding sections is the historical and philosophical case for how and why population health research is inseparable from social conceptions of health. Bell's insightful new book, *Health and Other Unassailable Values*, is right to take aim at the individualism and neo-liberalism of the so-called "New Public Health" of the 1970s (Bell 2017: 21–22). I disagree with the assertion that the public health community remains in that same era and mindset. While it is hard to gauge the degree of success of population health science and population health thinking, this chapter has argued that the historical path of population health science is rooted in a rejection of individualistic laissez-faire social ideology and remains opposed to it now. And, as noted in Chapter 1, population health science insights have been adopted in much of the public health science community as well. Chapter 3 will next elaborate that population health and individual health are more closely philosophically related than is typically recognized. It will do this by proposing a notion of social health that is suited for population health research and practice: *health as a life course trajectory of complete well-being in social context.*

The metaphysical, empirical, ethical, and methodological dimensions of health as social are intricately tied together by many threads that were gradually fastened over the course of the second half of the twentieth century. Not only does an ethical commitment to health as a social entity reinforce methods that fully embrace the social nature of health, but the reinforcement goes in both directions. In the analogous case of environmental science and policy,

Samuelsson and Rist have argued that engagement with stakeholders serves as a means of morally justifying environmental decisions—that is, good social methodology supports good social ethics (Samuelsson and Rist 2016). But the ethical argument for seeing health as a matter of empowerment and social justice is also tied to the gradual accumulation of evidence that disempowered people, as a matter of fact, live less healthy lives and that social context exerts a staggering amount of power over individuals' health. All of these connected threads reinforce the prescient wisdom of the original WHO assertion that health is social to its metaphysical core.

WHO's inconsistent record of addressing the social nature of health does not negate the laudability of its leadership in acknowledging it as such and showing similar intellectual leadership in facing the ethical and methodological consequences. For WHO, as with all others working in health promotion, the crux is coming to grips with the notion of health as a social phenomenon (not a property of atomistic individual humans abstracted from their social contexts) and designing all population health efforts accordingly.

Case study: The Standing Rock Sioux Water Protectors

In 2016 international headlines featured the dispute between the Standing Rock Sioux population and their supporters vs. the backers of a proposed Dakota Access Pipeline. The pipeline, now fully operational but still legally challenged, barely goes around the current borders of the Standing Rock Sioux Indian Reservation. But it travels through land that is vitally important to the Standing Rock Sioux for many reasons, in addition to the fact that the land rightfully belongs to the Sioux under an 1851 treaty that was violated by the US government

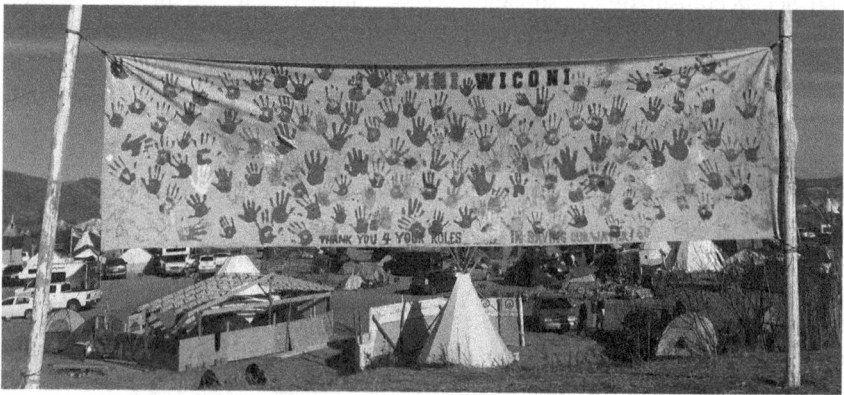

Figure 2.1 "mni wiconi banner" by Cathy Becker. A banner at the Oceti Sakowin camp protest site, depicting handprints of camp visitors and the protest slogan "mni wiconi" (water is life).

Source: Creative Commons Attribution 2.0 Generic license. www.flickr.com/photos/becker271/31015368944/.

(Whyte 2017). Applying this chapter's account of population health to the case helps to clarify the issues at stake, and reinforces the case of the anti-pipeline side, since population health considerations are sufficient reason to reject the pipeline, even setting aside the array of other compelling objections.

The concept of empowerment helps to trace the connections between the different dimension of population health's sociality (metaphysical, empirical, ethical, and methodological). Empowerment is both constitutive of a properly broad conception of health and it is also a prerequisite for effective promotion of health in multiple measures. Community well-being includes empowerment by definition; disempowerment causes unhealthy behaviors. That is, a person's ability to develop and pursue a healthy life plan is an important component of what it means to be healthy—those lacking that ability are less healthy by virtue of that inability, regardless of what diagnosable pathologies they may have. Separately, it is a matter of fact that a person who isn't empowered to develop and pursue a healthy life plan will almost certainly suffer ill effects in all manner of physiological health metrics (life expectancy, mobility, blood pressure, etc.).

Standing Rock Sioux health is metaphysically social. The Standing Rock Sioux report that that their culture and identity are inseparably tied to "the entirety of the land within the Tribe's traditional territory" (Standing Rock Sioux Tribe 2016). Hence:

> Destruction or damage to any one cultural resource, site, or landscape contributes to destruction of the Tribe's culture, history, and religion. Injury to the Tribe's cultural resources causes injury to the Tribe and its people.
>
> (Standing Rock Sioux Tribe 2016)

Such claims should be taken at face value, though the connection between water and Sioux well-being had been noted in scholarship before the Dakota Access Pipeline dispute arose. For example, "the word for health is 'wicozanni,' referring to 'life' and 'humans,' and includes 'mni,' for 'water'" (Satterfield et al. 2007: 7). More pointedly, the rallying cry of the Sioux Water Protectors is: *Mni wiconi!* [Water is life!], illustrated in Figure 2.1. That cry is more than a slogan, it is a distillation and declaration of a weighty metaphysical linkage in Sioux life between identity, culture, well-being, and control of water resources.

Standing Rock Sioux health is empirically social. The health aspects of the Dakota Access Pipeline dispute cannot be adequately understood without first understanding the historical and social context. The DAPL is just a recent manifestation in a centuries-long string of disempowering affronts to Sioux health. Even before the DAPL standoff started, Sioux County had the second highest rate of deaths before age 35 (Frohlich 2016). The flipside of health/well-being as social and malleable is that systematic social oppression—"structural violence," to use Paul Farmer's favored term from social medicine (Farmer 2003)—is that the malleability can be twisted into catastrophic social harms. For example, in a report on the epidemic of violence against native women in the US, even the Department of Justice felt compelled to acknowledge the literature partly attributing the violence to the repetition of the power dynamics that defined colonial violence: abusive paternalistic authority and domination (Bachman et al. 2008).

Standing Rock Sioux health is ethically inseparable from social empowerment. The ethical and the methodological aspects of Sioux health are closely related, since the imperative to pursue health through empowerment (avoiding disempowerment) and the need to carefully choose contextually appropriate methodologies are both especially pressing when the population being served is living under the enduring oppression of colonialism. These issues will return in the case study examined in Chapter 3, on Aboriginal Australians' health. Ranco et al. illustrate that questions of resource management in tribal settings are inseparable from ethical issues of power and metaphysical questions of the definition of health (Ranco et al. 2011). They stress that there is a dual challenge of both protecting health-related resources (e.g., Sioux water resources) and also ensuring that the methods used to protect the resources are themselves under the control of tribes, "using tribally-derived regulatory-cultural approaches" (Ranco et al. 2011: 229). Oppression begets oppression.

Standing Rock Sioux health research and health promotion must engage with health as a social phenomenon. Marmot's UN Commission on Social Determinants of Health agrees with Ranco et al.'s assessment that, methodologically, health promotion in indigenous populations must be under the control of those populations:

> How the Declaration on the Rights of Indigenous Peoples is operationalized for health and health equity within different sociopolitical contexts will require careful consideration, *led by Indigenous Peoples.*
>
> (Commission on Social Determinants of Health 2008: 160, emphasis added)

Equitably promoting population health of indigenous populations requires careful tailoring of research and interventions. Most importantly, the tailoring process itself needs to be put in the hands of members of those populations. Just as Ranco et al. point out the close relationship between the ethical and methodological aspects of health in American Indian environmental health, they similarly show the close links between the ethical and methodological. The settler–indigenous interactions between the Standing Rock Sioux and the US government show the vital importance of instituting methodologies of interaction, learning, and cultural exchange that embody respect and equity. To do otherwise is to repeat the ethically abhorrent power dynamics of colonialism.

Colonialism robbed the Standing Rock Sioux of many of their metaphysically and empirically vital health resources, including much of their land. Health promotion efforts in indigenous communities constantly run the risk of further oppressing indigenous epistemologies/knowledges and health valuation systems even when they attempt to help the communities. Most notably, to claim that toxic pollution from a potential oil spill is the *only* type of health harm at stake in DAPL opposition is to oppress the Standing Rock Sioux, for whom the linkage between water, land, health, religion, culture, and well-being is a reality of lived experience. In light of the above, it is crucial to see that a strict biomedical model-based understanding of health is incapable of accounting for the full range of health harms that the Dakota Access Pipeline inflicts on the Standing Rock Sioux population. In the case of the Dakota Access Pipeline, the harms are more than just the potential effects for toxin-induced pathologies via an oil spill. The toxicity of petroleum from oil spills is shockingly under-researched and the existing data shows the pathological effects remain unclear in scope and severity (Aguilera et al. 2010). Other harms to Standing Rock Sioux holistic (and socially contingent) health/well-being are far more immediate and unambiguous, so long as one's health concept does not put blinders on them that prevent them from seeing them. Moreover, the 1851 Treaty of Fort Laramie language insisting that the Sioux retain rights to hunting and fishing can be read as attempts to ensure dietary and health autonomy (1904). Instead, the land was taken away and now also one of the key waterways for the tribe's land (its full rightful land and the remnants left to it now). These are health harms. And so are the disempowering processes that performed those harms—as the Ottawa Charter reminds us, health and empowerment are two sides of the same coin (World Health Organization 1986).

Methodologies for engaging with the Standing Rock Sioux and their resistance to DAPL must be anti-colonial—decolonial (Spice 2016). Colonial power dynamics preclude ethical implementation of participatory health research and intervention by subverting the culture and governance of the colonized. As Allard illustrates, the Sioux political structures began as impositions, not community consent.

> Our traditional leaders were forced aside by the Indian Reorganization Act of 1936, when federal authorities forced the establishment of tribal councils on the reservations. This is a colonial system of government with no basis in Lakota/Dakota/Nakota culture or teachings.
>
> (Allard 2017)

Often acting subtly, "settler patriarchy destabilizes Indigenous political systems by subverting the traditional leadership of Indigenous women and non-binary people" to the point that "some Indigenous men" have begun claiming that the newly sexist gender roles are the traditional roles (Whyte and Meissner 2018). Again, disempowerment constitutes a health/well-being harm per se, instigates cascades of further harms (recall: "Beliefs in the effectiveness (or lack of it) of one's own actions are both learned, and reinforced by one's social position (Evans and Stoddart 1990: 1357)."), and disrupts communities' capacity to make equitable collective decisions about how to participate in health research and interventions.

It is sadly fitting to end on the case of Standing Rock Sioux health because the following chapter, on the nature of health, will advocate for an understanding of health as a life course, a trajectory rather than a state or process at a moment in time. Standing Rock Sioux health, much like the health of Aboriginal Australians, as explored in the next chapter's case study, reflects a particular set of health effects, intergenerational trauma, which must be understood with a temporally extended notion of health (Pember 2016).

Works cited

(1904) Treaty of Fort Laramie with the Sioux, etc. In: Kappler, C. J. (ed.) *Indian Affairs: Laws and Treaties.* Washington, DC: Government Printing Office, 594–596.

Aguilera, F., Méndez, J., Pásaro, E. and Laffon, B. (2010) Review on the effects of exposure to spilled oils on human health. *Journal of Applied Toxicology* 30, 291–301.

Allard, L. B. (2017) To save the water, we must break the cycle of colonial trauma. Available at: http://sacredstonecamp.org/blog/2017/2/4/to-save-the-water-we-must-break-the-cycle-of-colonial-trauma.

Amundson, R. (2005) Disability, Ideology, and Quality of Life. In: Wasserman, D., Bickenbach, J. and Wachbroit, R. (eds) *Quality of Life and Human Difference. Genetic Testing, Health Care and Disability.* Cambridge: Cambridge University Press, 101–120.

Bachman, R., Zaykowski, H., Kallmyer, R., et al. (2008) *Violence against American Indian and Alaska Native Women and the Criminal Justice Response: What is Known.* Washington, DC: National Institute of Justice.

Bell, K. (2017) *Health and Other Unassailable Values: Reconfigurations of Health, Evidence and Ethics.* London: Routledge.

Berridge, V. (2002) The Black Report and the health divide. *Contemporary British History* 16, 131–172.

Black, D., Morris, J., Smith, C. and Townsend, P. (1980) *Inequalities in Health: Report of a Research Working Group on Inequalities in Health.* London: Department of Health and Social Security.

Boorse, C. (1975) On the distinction between disease and illness. *Philosophy and Public Affairs* 5, 49–68.

Boorse, C. (1977) Health as a theoretical concept. *Philosophy of Science* 44, 542–573.

Boorse, C. (2014) A second rebuttal on health. *Journal of Medicine and Philosophy* 39, 683–724.

Burke, T. B. (2017) Choosing accommodations: Signed language interpreting and the absence of choice. *Kennedy Institute of Ethics Journal* 27, 267–299.

Campbell, S. M. and Stramondo, J. A. (2017) The complicated relationship of disability and well-being. *Kennedy Institute of Ethics Journal* 27, 151–184.

Carel, H. and Kidd, I. J. (2014) Epistemic injustice in healthcare: A philosophical analysis. *Medicine, Health Care and Philosophy* 17, 529–540.

Catford, J. (2011) Ottawa 1986: Back to the future. *Health Promotion International* 26, ii163–ii167.

Centers for Disease Control and Prevention. (2015) *Health in All Policies.* Available at: www.cdc.gov/policy/hiap/resources/.

Chetty, R., Stepner, M., Abraham, S., et al. (2016) The association between income and life expectancy in the United States, 2001–2014. *Journal of the American Medical Association* 315, 1750–1766.

Committee on Educating Health Professionals to Address the Social Determinants of Health. (2016) *A Framework for Educating Health Professionals to Address the Social Determinants of Health*. Washington, DC: National Academies Press.

Commission on Social Determinants of Health. (2008) *Closing the Gap in a Generation: Health Equity Through Action on the Social Determinants of Health*. Geneva: World Health Organization.

Daniels, N. (2006) Equity and population health: Toward a broader bioethics agenda. *Hastings Center Report* 36, 22–35.

Diez Roux, A. V. (2016) On the distinction—or lack of distinction—between population health and public health. *American Journal of Public Health* 106, 619–620.

Dunn, J. R. and Hayes, M. V. (1999) Toward a lexicon of population health. *Canadian Journal of Public Health* 90, S7–S10.

Elder, G. H., Kirkpatrick Johnson, M. and Crosnoe, R. (2003) The Emergence and Development of Life Course Theory. In: Mortimer, J. T. and Shanahan, M. J. (eds) *Handbook of the Life Course*. New York: Kluwer Academic, 3–19.

Evans, R. G. and Stoddart, G. L. (1990) Producing health, consuming health care. *Social Science and Medicine* 31, 1347–1363.

Evans, R. G., Barer, M. L., Hertzman, C., et al. (2010) Why are some books important (and others not)? *Canadian Journal of Public Health* 101, 433–435.

Evans, R. G., Barer, M. L. and Marmor, T. R. (1994) *Why Are Some People Healthy and Others Not? The Determinants of Health of Populations*. New York: Aldine De Gruyter.

Farmer, P. (2003) *Pathologies of Power: Health, Human Rights, and the New War on the Poor*. Berkeley, CA: University of California Press.

Freudenberg, N. and Tsui, E. (2014) Evidence, power, and policy change in community-based participatory research. *American Journal of Public Health* 104, 11–14.

Fricker, M. (2007) *Epistemic Injustice: Power and the Ethics of Knowing*. New York: Oxford University Press.

Frohlich, T. C. (2016) *37 Counties Where People Die Young*. Online news site, July 19, 2016: http://247wallst.com/special-report/2016/07/19/37-counties-where-people-die-young/9/.

Galea, S. (2018) *Healthier: Fifty Thoughts on the Foundations of Population Health*. New York: Oxford University Presss.

Granda, E. (2004) A qué llamamos salud colectiva, hoy? *Revista Cubana de Salud Pública* 30.

Granda, E. (2008) Algunas reflexiones a los veinticuatro años de la ALAMES. *Medicina Social* 3, 217–225.

House, J. S. (2015) *Beyond Obamacare: Life, Death, and Social Policy*. New York: Russell Sage Foundation.

International Conference on Primary Health Care. (1978) Declaration of Alma-Ata. Alma-Ata, Kazakhstan.

Irwin, A. and Scali, E. (2007) Action on the social determinants of health: A historical perspective. *Global Public Health* 2, 235–256.

Irwin, A. and Scali, E. (2010) Action on the Social Determinants of Health: Learning from Previous Experiences. *Social Determinants of Health Discussion Paper 1 (Debates)*. Geneva: World Health Organization.

James, J. E. (2015) *The Health of Populations: Beyond Medicine*. New York: Academic Press.

Keyes, K. M. and Galea, S. (2016) *Population Health Science*. New York: Oxford University Press.

Kickbusch, I. (2003) The contribution of the World Health Organization to a new public health and health promotion. *American Journal of Public Health* 93, 383–388.

Kickbusch, I. (2007) Health governance: The health society. In McQueen, D. V. and Kickbusch, I. (eds) *Health and Modernity*. New York: Springer, 144–161.

Krieger, N. (2011) *Epidemiology and the People's Health: Theory and Context*. New York: Oxford University Press.

Krieger, N. and Birn, A.-E. (1998) A vision of social justice as the foundation of public health: Commemorating 150 years of the spirit of 1848. *American Journal of Public Health* 88, 1603–1606.

Krueger, J. (2015) Theoretical health and medical practice. *Philosophy of Science* 82, 491–508.

Labonté, R., Polanyi, M., Muhajarine, N., et al. (2005) Beyond the divides: Towards critical population health research. *Critical Public Health* 15, 5–17.

Lalonde, M. (1974) *A New Perspective on the Health of Canadians*. Ottawa, Canada: Health and Welfare Canada.

Link, B. G. and Phelan, J. (1995) Social conditions as fundamental causes of disease. *Journal of Health and Social Behavior* 35, 80–94.

Link, B. G. and Phelan, J. C. (2002) McKeown and the idea that social conditions are fundamental causes of disease. *American Journal of Public Health* 92, 730–732.

Long, A. F. (1997) The Leeds Declaration: Three years on—a symbol or a catalyst for change? *Critical Public Health* 7, 73–81.

MacDonald, S. E., Newburn-Cook, C. V., Allen, M. and Reutter, L. (2013) Embracing the population health framework in nursing research. *Nursing Inquiry* 20, 30–41.

Marmot, M. (2004) *The Status Syndrome: How Social Standing Affects Our Health and Longevity*. New York: Henry Holt and Company.

Marmot, M. and Brunner, E. (2005) Cohort profile: The Whitehall II study. *International Journal of Epidemiology* 34, 251–256.

Marmot, M. G., Shipley, M. J. and Rose, G. (1984) Inequalities in death—specific explanations of a general pattern? *The Lancet* 323, 1003–1006.

McGovern, L., Miller, G. and Hughes-Cromwick, P. (2014) Health policy brief: The relative contribution of multiple determinants to health outcomes. *Health Affairs* 123, 1–8.

McHugh, N. A. (2015) *The Limits of Knowledge: Generating Pragmatist Feminist Cases for Situated Knowing*. Albany, NY: SUNY Press.

McKee, M., Stuckler, D., Dorner, T. and Paget, D. Z. (2016) *The Vienna Declaration*. Utrecht: European Public Health Association.

McKeown, T. (1976) *The Role of Medicine: Dream, Mirage, or Nemesis*. London: Nuffield Provincial Hospitals Trust.

Mittelmark, M. B., Sagy, S., Eriksson, M., et al. (2017) *The Handbook of Salutogenesis*. Cham, Switzerland: Springer.

Pember, M. A. (2016) *Intergenerational Trauma: Understanding Natives' Inherited Pain*. Indian Country Today Media Network.

Potvin, L. (2007) Managing Uncertainty Through Participation. In: McQueen, D. V. and Kickbusch, I. (eds) *Health and Modernity: The Role of Theory in Health Promotion*. New York: Springer.

Potvin, L. and Jones, C. M. (2011) Twenty-five years after the Ottawa Charter: The critical role of health promotion for public health. *Canadian Journal of Public Health* 102, 244–248.

Ranco, D. J., O'Neill, C. A., Donatuto, J. and Harper, B. L. (2011) Environmental justice, American Indians and the cultural dilemma: Developing environmental management for tribal health and well-being. *Environmental Justice* 4, 221–230.

Reid, L. (2015) Answering the empirical challenge to arguments for universal health coverage based in health equity. *Public Health Ethics* 9, 231–243.

Rose, G. (1992) *The Strategy of Preventive Medicine*. New York: Oxford University Press.

Saini, V., Garcia-Armesto, S., Klemperer, D., et al. (2017) Drivers of poor medical care. *The Lancet* 390, 178–190.

Salomon, J. A. and Murray, C. J. (2002) A Conceptual Framework for Understanding Adaptation, Coping and Adjustment in Health State Evaluations. *Summary Measures of Population Health: Concepts, Ethics, Measurement and Applications.* Geneva: World Health Organization, 619–626.

Samuelsson, L. and Rist, L. (2016) Stakeholder participation as a means to produce morally justified environmental decisions. *Ethics, Policy & Environment* 19, 76–90.

Satterfield, D. W., Shield, J. E., Buckley, J. and Alive, S. T. (2007) So that the people may live (Hecel Lena Oyate Ki Nipi Kte): Lakota and Dakota elder women as reservoirs of life and keepers of knowledge about health protection and diabetes prevention. *Journal of Health Disparities Research and Practice* 1, 1–28.

Secretary's Task Force on Black and Minority Health. (1985) Report of the Secretary's Task Force on Black and Minority Health. Washington, DC: US Department of Health and Human Services.

Shanahan, M. J., Mortimer, J. T. and Johnson, M. K. (2016) Introduction: Life Course Studies—Trends, Challenges, and Future Directions. In: Shanahan, M. J., Mortimer, J. T. and Johnson, M. K. (eds) *Handbook of the Life Course*. New York: Springer, 1–23.

Smocovitis, V. B. (1996) *Unifying Biology: The Evolutionary Synthesis and Evolutionary Biology*. Princeton, NJ: Princeton University Press.

Spice, A. (2016) Interrupting industrial and academic extraction on native land. *Hot Spots, Cultural Anthropology website.* Available at: https://culanth.org/fieldsights/1021-interrupting-industrial-and-academic-extraction-on-native-land.

Standing Rock Sioux Tribe. (2016) *Complaint for Declaratory and Injunctive Relief: Case 1:16-cv-01534.* Available at: http://earthjustice.org/sites/default/files/files/3154%201%Complaint.pdf.

Szreter, S. (2003) The population health approach in historical perspective. *American Journal of Public Health* 93, 421–431.

Szreter, S. (2005) *Health and Wealth*. Rochester, NY: University of Rochester Press.

The Lancet Editors. (1994) Population health looking upstream. *The Lancet* 343, 429–432.

Waitzkin, H. (2007) Political Economic Systems and the Health of Populations: Historical Thought and Current Directions. In: Galea, S. (ed.) *Macrosocial Determinants of Population Health*. New York: Springer Science Business Media, 105–138.

Wallerstein, N. and Duran, B. (2010) Community-based participatory research contributions to intervention research: The intersection of science and practice to improve health equity. *American Journal of Public Health* 100, S40–S46.

Whitehead, M. (1987) *The Health Divide: Inequalities in Health in the 1980s*. London: Health Education Council.

WHO Regional Office for Europe. (1988) Priority Research for Health for All. *European Health for All Series*. Copenhagen: World Health Organization.

Whyte, K. and Meissner, S. N. (2018) Theorizing Indigeneity, Gender, and Settler Colonialism. In: Taylor, P., Alcoff, L. M. and Anderson, L. (eds) *Routledge Companion to the Philosophy of Race*. New York: Routledge.

Whyte, K. P. (2017) The Dakota Access Pipeline, environmental injustice, and US colonialism. *Red Ink* 19, 154–169.

Working Group on Healthy Municipalities and Communities. (2005) *Healthy Municipalities, Cities and Communities: Evaluation Recommendations for Policymakers in the Americas*. Washington, DC: Pan American Health Organization.

World Health Organization. (1946) Official Records of the World Health Organization. *International Health Conference*. New York: United Nations.

World Health Organization. (1981) Global Strategy for Health for All by the Year 2000. Geneva: World Health Organization.

World Health Organization. (1986) Ottawa Charter for Health Promotion. Ottawa, ON: World Health Organization.

Yadavendu, V. K. (2014) *Shifting Paradigms in Public Health*. New Delhi: Springer India.

3 Health as a life course trajectory of complete well-being in social context

Introduction: the many debates over health's meaning

"Population health science" has no single narrow meaning, but the core of this new science, approach, framework, paradigm—whatever it may be—is the goal of reconstructing the theory and practice of how to promote the health of populations, in reaction to the lessons learned from twentieth-century public health and healthcare. So, it should be no surprise that this ambitious reconstruction process has repeatedly found itself struggling with the question of what we should take the meaning of health to be in this new population health science enterprise. In this chapter, I defend a new health concept, an adaptation of the World Health Organization's social concept of health, described in Chapter 2, combining that concept of health with Life Course Theory. Life Course Theory is an interdisciplinary theory of human health and development that frames human life as a socially embedded trajectory lasting the entire lifespan. In defending my new concept of health, I explain that it is designed to serve as a sort of pluralistic meta-concept (a toolbox for health concepts, not the tool itself), compatible with a wide range of health concepts and health assessment methods.

The standard dichotomy in philosophical debates over the nature of health is between non-evaluative vs. evaluative definitions, disputing whether health is an objective fact of the world or something that requires subjective normative judgment about the goodness and badness of certain conditions (Humber and Almeder 2010; Carel and Cooper 2014). Coggon helpfully suggests that we also take into account two additional dichotomies: positive vs. negative health concepts (disputing whether health is the positive presence of something or simply the absence of disease), and internal vs. external health concepts (disputing whether health is the sort of thing that must be measured by external observers or reported by each person living with that health experience) (Coggon 2012: 11–20). This chapter will not seek to fully resolve these and other related disputes. I think that Amartya Sen is on the right track when he favors internalism for its humanistic recognition of health as an experience while also acknowledging that sometimes externalism is required to help us take a step back and recognize how social conditions shape perceptions of health (Sen 2004). But, in this chapter, I advocate a pluralistic meta-conception of health that is designed to be only as narrow as needed to guide health promotion efforts. The most controversial stance I take within the landscape of philosophy of medicine's debates over the meaning of health is in my advocacy for a positive conception of health. This is in keeping with the WHO positive conception of which, that includes the absence of disease as one set of ingredients for health but also requires the presence of well-being.

The most prominent advocate of holistic health concepts in the philosophy of medicine community is Lennart Nordenfelt. Over his career he has offered many arguments in favor of holistic health over competing health concepts. Given my philosophical methodological orientation toward respecting and seeking to learn from the knowledge of non-philosophers, I am particularly interested in Nordenfelt's contention that holistic health concepts are already ubiquitous outside of philosophy.

> I claim that there is a set of related conceptions of holistic health embedded in ordinary language. These conceptions are influential, not only in common discourse but also in public debate, in health promotion, and in many sectors of healthcare.
>
> (Nordenfelt 2016: 212)

This chapter offers an addendum to this contention by arguing that life course theory is also widely used outside of philosophy, and that much can be learned from its prevalence, just like we can learn much from the prevalence of holistic health-thinking. I synthesize holistic health-thinking and life course health-thinking, by adapting WHO's holistic concept of health to more explicitly incorporate the insights of a life course model of health.

This chapter's content is foremost guided by a concern for the "real world" repercussions of health concepts—applicability to health science practices, relevance to human well-being, the looming dangers of cultural imperialism, and related concerns about the consequences of advocating for health concepts. I only offer a single overarching—though pluralistic—concept of health because I think it is of practical value. In this book of outward-looking and engaged philosophy, I take a philosophical problem to be pressing if engaging in philosophical analysis and discourse would be a plausible means of serving the interests of non-philosophers. As I will revisit in Chapter 7, I concur with Lemoine (2013), Schwartz (2014), and Griffiths and Matthewson (2016) that the problem of defining health should not be trying to uncover the "true" meaning of health, but more like the process of doing concept "explication" in the tradition of Carnap and Quine—philosophers should strive to make health concepts more illuminating and useful.

Life course theory

Life course theory and population health science both have tangled historical roots (see Chapter 2) (Elder et al. 2003; Kindig and Stoddart 2003). It seems that the two lines of research arose independently out of innovations stretching back to at least the first half of the twentieth century, and that each began exponentially increasing its appearances in published literature beginning in roughly the mid-1990s (Shanahan et al. 2016). After emerging in parallel, they are now partially converging. Life course theory is now a mature general theory for the study of human lives. Like population health science, it advocates for an interdisciplinary theoretical approach offered as a corrective to the failures of the previous researchers (see Chapter 2). In the case of life course theory, it was a reaction to the problem that sociologists of the early twentieth century had been too disinterested in longitudinal aspects of human life and too blind to the power of social contexts (which also change over time) (Elder et al. 2003: 3–4). Life Course Theory emerged out of a rejection of a deep dissatisfaction of the view of human life offered by earlier scholarship: richly detailed snapshots of people that still only captured moments in time, snapshots so single-mindedly focused on their human subjects that the background was left blurry. By contrast, Life Course Theory replaces single zoomed-in snapshots with video or photo montages observing people over long periods of time, zoomed out to ensure that subjects are seen inside their surrounding environments. Life Course Theory is far too wide-ranging to fully summarize here (Elder et al. 2003); I will extract only two of the key principles offered by the theory.

The first lesson I will extract from Life Course Theory is the warning to avoid assessment of health at a single moment in time—it must be assessed with respect to a developmental trajectory that occurs over time. Even when philosophers construe health as a process, the time component is typically left in background or limited to a snippet of time, such as the course of an infection (see discussion in Smart 2014). The second lesson I will extract is that individuals' health develops through dynamic relationships with the healths of their population and their social-environmental contexts. This echoes Chapter 2's historical account of the gradual recognition of health as a social phenomenon.

Keyes and Galea surmise the importance of Life Course Theory for population health science when they offer the following as one of their nine "foundational principles" of population health science: "The causes of population health are multilevel, accumulate throughout the life course, and are embedded in dynamic interpersonal relationships" (Keyes and Galea 2016: xiii).[1] As population health scholar Onyebuchi Arah describes in a 2009 philosophy article attempting to bridge population health theory and philosophical understanding of health: individual health and population health dynamically co-develop over time.

> Neither individuals nor collectives can be understood in only cross-sectional, one-time views ... collectives age across generations of its members, evolving and defining and being defined through cumulative and adaptive experiences, events, and history.
>
> (Arah 2009: 240)

A Life Course Theory perspective on health as a lifelong trajectory clarifies how health is deeply embedded in social processes. Alternative concepts of health that put less emphasis on health's longitudinal aspects are limited in their capacity to engage with the accumulated mutual dynamics of the individual and their social context.

Life course lesson 1: health is best understood as a lifelong phenomenon, not in time slices

> Concepts of health and models of health promotion have long struggled when contending with diseases that emerge very gradually, such as chronic diseases.
>
> (Fuller 2017)

Such diseases are hard to pin down with the language of physiological processes or discrete bodily states when the processes and states change drastically over time (e.g., the gradual transition from pre-diabetic insulin resistance to the multitude of Type 2 diabetes symptoms), though it is possible to account for them this way (Fuller 2017; Smart 2014). Even before it became widely accepted that chronic diseases should be global health promotion priorities, Corbin and Strauss offered a new model of chronic disease that pushed back against the perceived limitations of biomedical model accounts of chronic diseases that represented the diseases as only physiological states and processes. They instead proposed the Chronic Illness Trajectory Framework (Corbin and Strauss 1988):

> under which, a chronic illness is viewed as a serious disease affecting a person's mental, emotional and social well-being, and a trajectory is a course of illness over time, together with the actions taken by patients, families and health professionals to manage or shape the course of this illness.
>
> (Morales-Asencio et al. 2016: 123)

As will be elaborated in the next section, this notion of a temporally extended *trajectory* of disease complements a social understanding of disease, in which the processes of disease are experienced and responded to by both patients and the people around them. For the moment I am drawing attention to the temporal aspect of the model, including the trajectory metaphor's representation of health/disease moving through time not as a branching series of mechanisms and processes, but instead as an object on a path, with a path behind it and a combination of direction and momentum that together resist attempts to redirect it. The case of atherosclerosis, cholesterol blockage in the arteries, serves to illustrate the benefits of understanding health as a life course trajectory.

Atherosclerosis has long been a point of difficulty and contention for philosophers of medicine, as it is a condition that exists on a spectrum in all people; everyone's arteries have at least some cholesterol/lipid plaque and inflammation from it (Boorse 1977; Giroux 2015). This is the source of a series of questions about normality, appropriate comparison/reference populations, etc. (Boorse 1977; Giroux 2015; Fuller 2017). Any specific health concept will struggle with at least some number of outlier cases, but no worthy health concept can afford to fumble the atherosclerosis case. The cardiovascular diseases caused by atherosclerotic inflammation and plaque accumulation in the arteries are an enormous source of global morbidity and mortality. In the 195 countries monitored by the Global Burden of Disease Study, 21.3 percent of the deaths in 2015 were due to just two of the diseases caused by atherosclerosis, ischemic heart disease and ischemic stroke (GBD 2015 Mortality and Causes of Death Collaborators 2016: 1484, 1488). Life course thinking and a temporally extended trajectory understanding of health offer a way forward, but require some serious conceptual and practical shifts.

In light of the need to develop more effective treatment models for atherosclerotic disease, in 2013 the American College of Cardiology and American Heart Association released new guidelines for cholesterol management to prioritize patients' life course trajectories when treating atherosclerotic cardiovascular disease (Stone et al. 2014). The guidelines prioritize the assessment of whether a patient's trajectory is heading toward harm from a major cardiovascular event in the foreseeable future, a radical shift from earlier treatment guidelines' focus on whether a patient's LDL ("bad") cholesterol level is high enough to currently qualify as a pathological disease state meriting treatment via a statin drug (Finkel and Duffy 2015; Stone et al. 2014; Goff et al. 2013). The old question for the physician assessing whether to begin a treatment regime such as a statin drug (e.g., Lipitor) was: "Are this patient's LDL cholesterol levels, and the associated lipid plaque in their arteries, elevated enough to require drug therapy?" The new question, after the 2013 ACC/AHA shift became: "Based on available knowledge about this patient (age, tobacco use, cholesterol levels, etc.), how likely are they to have a heart attack or other major cardiovascular episode in the foreseeable future?" The ACC/AHA switch to a life course perspective has two arguments in its favor. First, atherosclerosis accumulates over very long periods of time:

> extensive epidemiological, pathological, and basic science data indicate that the development of atherosclerosis … occurs over decades and is related to long-term and cumulative exposure to causal, modifiable risk factors. Thus, a life-course perspective on risk assessment and prevention must be taken, especially among younger individuals.
>
> (Goff et al. 2013: 2945)

The second practical reason for shifting to a life course perspective is that it refocuses attention on the long-term risk of harm, rather than focusing on reducing the current cholesterol level into an acceptable range (Finkel and Duffy 2015). But Life Course Theory's contribution to an updated health concept is more than an admonition to think long-term or think about prevention. Rather, it makes long-term trajectory the subject of intervention—a patient's current level of arterial plaque is demoted to a secondary consideration, only relevant as it relates to the predicted risk of a major cardiovascular episode. As previously mentioned in the Chronic Illness Trajectory Framework (Corbin and Strauss 1988), it is best to pair a long-term view of health with a view that foregrounds the complex dynamics between individuals, populations, environments, and general social contexts.

Life course lesson 2: population health and individual health are best understood as co-developing dynamically

The standard distinction between individual health and population health begins to dissolve when one adopts a life course perspective. As Arah explains:

> a person's health cannot be seen in isolation but must be placed in the rich contextual web such as the socioeconomic circumstances and other health determinants of where they were conceived, born, bred, and how they shaped and were shaped by their environment and communities.
>
> (Arah 2009: 235)

The trajectory of the individual and the trajectory of the social context are inextricably linked, and so any attempt to assess one will necessarily involve the other. As surmised by bioethicist Thomas May and colleagues, the move toward a population health management approach, "collapses traditional distinctions between clinical medicine and public health by emphasizing the symbiotic relationship between individual patients and broader populations" (May et al. 2017: 167).

By taking a longitudinal view of life and health, we make it far easier to see the dynamics between individual health and population health. As Chapter 2 describes at length, health is thoroughly social. As such, attempts to split individual health from population health are dubious at best. Along similar lines, Krueger criticizes Boorse's biomedical/Biostatistical model for building individual health from the bottom-up—a complete set of disease-free tissues constitutes a healthy person (Krueger 2015).[2] In Boorse's account, populations serve as comparison classes for judging the statistically normal body part activities that define a healthy body—other features of social contexts fade into the background. Moving the dynamics of social life from background to foreground allows us to recognize and intervene upon the synergies that mutually reinforce good health or poor health; a patient is not a collection of functioning/malfunctioning organic machinery floating in a vacuum.

Take the much-publicized problem of unhealthful fast-food restaurants' popularity among wealthy nations, particularly in subpopulations with lower socioeconomic status. On the one hand, it may be tempting to try to paternalistically solve the problem of fast-food consumption by having governments ban these restaurants. On the other hand, one might also be tempted to put in place an education campaign (inevitably meager and underfunded compared to fast-food advertising) and then place all responsibility on individuals who fail to adopt healthier habits. Either of those options only recognizes a one-way causal arrow from population/environment to the individual within it. Individual-population dietary health dynamics are a two-way street. A person's level of desire for fast food is shaped by a combination of factors operating over the complete life course, from accumulated taste preferences to advertising, and acting on those tastes by buying fast food reinforces the fast-food market. For example, in the US, Black children and rural children are disproportionately targeted for fast-food advertising (Ohri-Vachaspati et al. 2015), which causes individuals within these populations to increasingly desire these foods and hence drives the disproportionate consumption of fast food in these populations. Accordingly, recent research on obesity interventions suggests that the most promising way forward is to recognize the complexity of individual dietary health choices/behaviors (Backholer et al. 2014). The most promising avenue is to recognize that individual people are both agents of action and change within their social contexts and also affected by those social contexts (Backholer et al. 2014).

Having briefly extracted two recent lessons from life course theory—health is a lifelong trajectory and health is a dynamic interplay between individuals–populations/environments—I will now return to the 1946 World Health Organization concept of health discussed in Chapter 2 and synthesize it with these two contributions from Life Course Theory. First, it is crucial to examine why the definition has received so much criticism, most of all from philosophers. The WHO definition has often served as a foil for those seeking to contrast their own health concepts with the broad WHO concept. Such criticism is misguided.

The World Health Organization's definition of health, not what it seems

The 1946 Constitution of the World Health Organization includes a definition of health. "Health is a state of complete physical, mental and social well-being and not merely the absence of disease or infirmity" (World Health Organization 1946: 100). That definition remains a source of dispute. The two key objections leveled against the WHO definition are that it foolishly muddles the concepts of health and well-being, and that WHO does not even use its own definition of health (perhaps because of the purported health–well-being muddle). Understanding why these critiques are misguided helps to make it clearer what makes the WHO definition a suitable core for my new pluralistic health concept.

Norman Daniels sees no fundamental incompatibility between the study of social determinants of health and the use of a naturalistic absence-of-disease definition of health, and chastises WHO for undermining its own health promotion efforts by defining health as the positive presence of well-being:

> the WHO conception erroneously expands health to include nearly all of wellbeing, so it can no longer function as a limit notion. People who actually measure population health, such as epidemiologists, concentrate on departures from normal functioning.
>
> (Daniels 2006: 33)

Daniels is correct that there is no *prima facie* incommensurability between conceiving of health as absence of biological dysfunction and also acknowledging the power of social determinants of health. Echoing Daniels, Daniel Hausman dismisses the WHO definition for "conflat[ing] health and well-being, and, although it has never been formally repudiated, the World Health Organization does not rely on this definition in its attempts to measure health" (Hausman 2015: 18). The problem is that such departures from "normal functioning" only represent some of the ways that health can be harmed, such as in Chapter 2's case study of the Standing Rock Sioux and the Dakota Access Pipeline. The health harms of the pipeline include risks to the "normal functioning" of their bodies (e.g., the risk of oil spills), but the complete set of well-being harms includes more (e.g., the spiritual harms and identity harms). Standing Rock Sioux population health is catastrophically harmed by the Dakota Access Pipeline via affronts to their spiritual well-being and to the linkages between individual/community identity and the natural environment.

The concerns expressed by Daniels and Hausman are related to the objection that the WHO definition of health is too expansive because such a notion risks "the tyranny of health" (Callahan 1973). That is, a broad concept of health could allow medicine to grow hegemonic and claim all matters of well-being as being under its authority. Health promotion is already used all too readily by various biomedical authorities and lay supporters as an automatic policy justification (Bell 2017; Metzl and Kirkland 2010). For example, medical(ized social) surveillance of pregnant women's bodies is already oppressive (Kukla 2010). This is a very serious issue. Accordingly, Chapter 4 is devoted to defusing this concern, showing that concerns of health hegemony and the so-called "boundary problem" of what is/isn't a health matter both fail as objections to population health science's ambitiously broad agenda of looking in all corners of human social life for the causes and effects of health. The worry that such broad models of health necessarily lead to medical hegemony or tyranny (doctors expanding their social power, etc.) fails because population health science emphatically agrees that medicine is inappropriately powerful as an institution. Population health science is founded on a rejection of the idea that all health matters are automatically the domain of healthcare. Under a population health science philosophy, health may be everywhere in social life, but health governance ought to be participatory and empowering (see argument in Chapter 7, p. 170) and healthcare is only one of many sectors of society responsible for collaboratively and humbly seeking to advance health (see argument in Chapter 8, p. 187).

Anti-WHO definition critiques from applied population health scholars have largely focused on the problem of whether the WHO definition can be effectively operationalized for practical use. Evans and Stoddart's epochal 1990 population health science article devotes considerable space to reviewing the benefits and drawbacks of the WHO definition (Evans and Stoddart 1990). They praise the precision of the competing negative concept of health, while stressing that WHO's definition was left as a lonely "voice in the woods" after its writing (Evans and Stoddart 1990: 1348). In reply, Ronald Labonté—long a critical voice within the population health science community—chastised Evans and Stoddart's ambivalence toward WHO's positive concept of health, arguing that doing so tacitly perpetuates a "reductionist biomedical theory of health" (Labonté 1995: 166). Nash et al.'s 2016 textbook supports the WHO definition of health and laments its historical neglect (moreover: "now is the time to fully embrace the idea of health as a state of well-being, vitality, performance, and a high quality of life") (Edington et al. 2016: 386). Kindig, arguably population health thinking's most active popularizer, places the WHO definition alongside various other definitions of "health," in his glossary of population health key terms and the discussion thereof, while declining to decisively choose between the positive WHO concept vs. a negative concept (Kindig 2007: 142, 145). Perhaps best encapsulating the concerns of population health scholars, Young's textbook on population health praises the WHO definition for orienting practitioners to think about promoting the presence of health, rather than just focusing on disease treatment (this theme will return in Chapter 5's discussion of "salutogenesis" theory) (Young 2005: 3). Yet, he worries about its practicality and says the key is having an "'operational' definition" of health (Young 2005: 3).

I agree entirely with Young's point about the need to properly operationalize the WHO concept of health. However, I think Young and other skeptics have misread the WHO definition. The population health science community's reception of the WHO definition as philosophically appealing but practically lackluster leads to the next section of the chapter. Critics have mistaken what the WHO definition is and does: it outlines a *meta-concept* of health, a conceptual framework within which particular operational concepts of health can be specified for particular purposes in particular communities—the WHO definition is not an operational definition to be used in applied research or policy "off the shelf."

The WHO definition of health is not an operationalized tool for health assessment; it is a toolbox that guides the gathering of tools

The WHO definition of health is far too vague to be used as a technical term without modification. The definition simply states, "Health is a state of complete physical, mental and social well-being and not merely the absence of disease or infirmity" (World Health Organization 1946: 100). Much needs to be specified and adapted before use. Bickenbach's survey of the critiques of this "notorious" definition argues that it is insufficiently "susceptible to operationalization" (Bickenbach 2015: 961–962). Critics seem to infer that there is an implied addendum to the WHO definition, "… and this definition should be adopted without modification in health research and practice, and that health cannot include other elements in its holism, regardless of context." I see no reason to infer this. WHO traced out a definition of health—perhaps better described as a meta-concept of health, an outline of a class of health concepts—and left questions of operationalization to the legions of scholars and practitioners to follow. In other words, the question is not whether the WHO definition is the right *tool* for doing population health work; the question is whether the WHO definition is the right sort of *toolbox* for collecting tools for doing population health work. Is it the sort of toolbox that accommodates our current tools, and guides us toward collecting new tools to fill conspicuous gaps in the tool collection? As described below, limiting health to the absence of disease needlessly prevents us from considering health matters that seem overwhelmingly relevant to health. But, as signaled in the above critiques by Daniels and Hausman, defending the desirability of the WHO definition of health also requires rebutting the objection that is often paired with the first objection, the claim that WHO does not actually use its own definition.

As discussed in Chapter 2, Cold War-era US influence stifled the application of social concepts of health due to a combination of anti-socialist politics and technocratic idealism. But, in the 1990s the tide turned (Irwin and Scali 2007). I can think of no plainer evidence that the WHO concept is alive and well than pointing to the title of the official WHO Twelfth Programme of Work, the "high-level strategic vision for the work of WHO for the period 2014–2019": its title is *Not Merely the Absence of Disease* (World Health Organization 2014). In other words, attending to holistic well-being is not just some incidental component of WHO's plan of action for 2014–2019; it is the organizing principle of its work. Critics can continue objecting that WHO (and the global public health community for whom it serves as leader) ought not promote holistic well-being. But the charge that WHO and its network of public health workers *don't* do such work is simply wrong.

As a broad meta-concept of health, when the WHO definition is used it is not always obvious at first glance. Take, for example, the way that it serves as a basis for "reproductive health" research, going through a two-stage operationalization process to take it from the 1946 definition to population health practice (World Health Organization Regional Committee for Europe 2016: 25). The first step is adapting the WHO definition into a specific health concept suited to the relevant task—assessing and promoting global reproductive health.

> "Reproductive health is a state of complete physical, mental and social well-being and not merely the absence of disease or infirmity, *in all matters relating to the reproductive system and to its functions and processes.*"
> (International Conference on Population and Development 1994: 40, emphasis added)

This narrows the general WHO definition for application to reproductive health, the area of interests. The resulting definition is non-obvious, grounded in a holistic understanding of health, and hence concerned with more than just the absence of sexual/reproductive pathologies. This definition of reproductive health, according to WHO, "implies that people are able to have a satisfying and safe sex life and that they have the capability to reproduce and the freedom to decide if, when and how often to do so" (International Conference on Population and Development 1994: 40). Using this particular definition makes a pivotal difference in how we measure and intervene in population-level reproductive health. For instance, a population with low rates of diagnosable gynecological pathologies, but in which women are socially coerced to bear large numbers of children, has poor sexual and reproductive health. Under a biomedical concept of health, a negative concept, low rates of reproductive/sexual disease would automatically qualify that same population as relatively healthy and thus having a low priority in reproductive health efforts. WHO is right to assert that a reproductively healthy population is free from reproductive coercion; it strains credulity to say a population has good reproductive health if it is filled with women who are pregnant against their wills.

After the first step of adapting the WHO definition to reproductive health, WHO then performs the second step of operationalizing it in applied health assessment and health promotion ventures. One prominent way WHO is doing that now is through the joint UN-WHO program, Every Woman, Every Child. That program uses a life course model (of course!) to conceptualize the well-being of women as being practically inseparable from the health of children and adolescents due to the global prevalence of social and biological bonds through birth, childcare, etc. (Every Woman Every Child 2015). Accordingly, the program pushes for specific health interventions at important periods in the life course, including HIV screening/treatment in pregnant women, developing "school curricula" that "include elements to strengthen the self-esteem of girls and increase respect for girls among boys," along with strengthening laws and policies to prevent "violence against women and girls" across all periods of the life course (Every Woman Every Child 2015: 21, 61, 89). Since health is so socially contingent and linked to empowerment (see Chapter 2 on WHO's Ottawa Charter), the program urges: "encourage communities to participate in defining their health needs. Reorient health and development services in response" (Every Woman Every Child 2015: 61). The WHO definition provided the holistic toolbox, which constrained the size and shape of the compartment for the tools used to assess and promote reproductive health. That in turn led WHO to set specific reproductive goals and metrics, looking not just to HIV transmission and other standard biomedical pathologies but also holistic well-being matters, including education, self-esteem, respect, and institutional protections against violence.

Making room for health pluralisms: metaphysical, empirical, ethical, and methodological

Combining the lessons of the first and second halves of this chapter yields an update to WHO's 1946 health concept, an update I see as compatible with the original definition because the original definition offered a loose framework mainly characterized by the commitment to health as the positive presence of well-being in social context. I extend the WHO health concept over the life course, yielding a new definition of health: *health as a life course trajectory of complete well-being in social context*. I conceive of my variation on the WHO concept of health, like the original version, to be more akin to a toolbox than a tool itself. It is a very large toolbox that can fit a huge range of other tools in it. I do not propose this health meta-concept as the sole "correct" health concept. Instead, I offer it as the one that I judge to offer a worthy and non-obvious guiding framework for the many healths that exist in the diverse social world. There is no single universal capital-H "Health." While I offer a definition of health, I wish to nonetheless leave room for health pluralism in four different senses: metaphysically, empirically, ethically, and methodologically. These parallel Chapter 2's argument that there are four different senses of health-as-social.

Metaphysically, a *trajectory of complete well-being in social context* is pluralistic, but still takes a non-obvious stance. Different populations have different health ontologies—health (well-being) for the Standing Rock Sioux is fundamentally not the same thing as health for the settler US populations that surround them; among other reasons, the statuses of ancestral Sioux lands and waters are inseparable from their spirituality, culture, identity, and well-being. Non-Sioux in the same region can value entities such as Lake Oahe (which is now traversed by the pipeline), but harm to that body of water is only an instrumental harm—usurpation of, or damage to, Lake Oahe is not a harm per se to non-Sioux. Healths vary.

Philosophers of health continue to have valuable nuanced discourse over the metaphysics of health, such as whether it is best conceptualized as a capability (Ruger 2010), a meta-capability (a capability to have other capabilities), or perhaps an ability to reach one's "vital goals" (Nordenfelt 2016). I decline to insist on any of these additional metaphysics of health over and above what is already captured in my posited definition. I think the original WHO definition was right to leave room not only for a plurality of health experiences but also of health metaphysics. As noted in the Standing Rock Sioux case study, and as will be reiterated in the upcoming case study of Aboriginal Australian health, one essential component of equitable and empowering health promotion is respecting others' health concepts. To be clear, my account of health demands more than just respecting Sioux or Aboriginal Australian peoples' *beliefs* about health. Instead, my meta-concept of health demands that we recognize that diverse communities around the world have healths that genuinely *are* different. Health includes all of well-being and is inextricable from social context; well-beings in social contexts will vary widely because the features of well-being and social structures vary widely.

Empirical health pluralism follows quickly from the adoption of a holistic well-being concept of health. Well-being is a drastically different thing in different populations, reflecting the rather obvious fact that we have drastically different goals, priorities, sexual practices, occupations, climates, diets, spiritual and religious beliefs, and practices, etc. Again, Standing Rock Sioux well-being is, metaphysically, intimately tied to ancestral land and the waters therein. Given that health's meaning and components vary, it is rather obvious that these meanings would manifest empirically in a similar plurality of ways. In a sense, the metaphysical concept of health proposed by WHO is a response to the empirical fact that social contexts—and hence what it looks like to have well-being in those contexts—are diverse. In the face of the abundantly obvious fact that social life and social well-being varies enormously by population, WHO made the decision to embrace that and posit that there is a plurality of healths in the world, situated in the plurality of social experiences.

Ethically, it is unacceptable to impose a culturally incongruous health concept onto a population. A *life course trajectory of complete well-being in social context* foregrounds social context and history. It also intentionally declines to give some top-down decree of what complete well-being is. In the case of the Standing Rock Sioux, this means that fully applying my health concept would require researchers and policymakers to fully include Standing Rock Sioux people in the process of crafting a set of operationalized health assessment tools. Those tools should presumably include means of assessing the population's well-being in light of the land–water–spirituality–identity–health linkages in their social context. For example, future health assessments would likely be substantially enriched by gathering survey data about community members' perceptions of the accessibility and integrity of sacred waters and how this affects the intergenerational transmission of cultural knowledge and practices.

Methodologically, one can accept *health as a life course trajectory of complete well-being in social context* as the toolbox for health assessment, while fully accepting that most tools used for health assessment will have rather limited ranges of use. Work done under the aegis of any health concept routinely requires measuring only a subset of its components (e.g., measuring incidences of a single disease) (Hausman 2015). I offer the above health concept as a large toolbox that guides us as we collect a repertoire of health measurement and health promotion tools. Many or most tools in the toolbox will also be fully consistent with biomedical concepts of health, such as Boorse's Biostatistical Theory (Boorse 2014). One key contribution of my meta-concept is that it helps show us where there are gaps in our toolset. For example, it inclines a dietary health researcher to ask whether current data collection practices are adequate for gathering the longitudinal (life course) impacts of various diets, rather than just the short-term impacts on biomarkers such as plasma cholesterol levels.

While this chapter lacks the space to systematically contrast my meta-concept of health with every alternative concept or approach, it is worth taking a moment to address the "capabilities approach" to justice and well-being, which is different from my own but remains broadly compatible. This approach has risen to prominence in the global health equity literature thanks to overlapping efforts by Martha Nussbaum (2011), Amartya Sen (2005), Jennifer Prah Ruger (2010), Sridhar Venkatapuram (2011), and Madison Powers and Ruth Faden (2006), among others. Though variously specified by its proponents, it generally conceives of well-being as the presence of certain capabilities in each person, such as the capability to form social relationships with others. Venkatapuram contends that health is, in fact, a "meta-capability" that allows other human capabilities to operate (Venkatapuram 2011). He frames this position as an "extension" of Nordenfelt's earlier work on "health as the ability to reach one's vital goals" (Venkatapuram 2011). While my concept defers to the local social context in order to establish what "well-being" means in that context, I have no objection to the capabilities approach's list of ten positive traits as one way of specifying a broad social justice mandate to promote complete health and well-being. The health capabilities approach will feature again in Chapter 4's dispute with Powers and Faden's interpretation of the scope of public health and in Chapter 7's account of how population health science and health equity interrelate.

Conclusion: an updated health concept for an expansive population health mission

I argue that there is great value in conceiving of health fundamentally as the positive presence of well-being, and that there is great value in conceiving of that well-being as a trajectory that spans the entire life course. This account of *health as a life course trajectory of complete well-being in social context* is built upon the historical lessons outlined in Chapter 2. That chapter offered a historical account of the gradual recognition among population health experts that health is social: in its metaphysical nature, its empirical causal dynamics, its ethical considerations, and its methodological considerations.

There are two related Life Course Theory insights components that my definition of health incorporates: (1) health should be understood as a long-term trajectory, rather than a momentary state or short-term set of discrete processes, and (2) health should be understood within a dynamic social relationship between individuals and the population–environmental–social contexts in which they reside. These two features are philosophically complementary, since a longitudinal view of health allows one to better see the causal push and pull between individuals and their surroundings; conversely, recognizing that there are such dynamic relationships leads to the next intuitive step of taking a long-term view of health in order to observe the processes and effects of those dynamic relationships.

This chapter updates and defends the WHO concept of health, arguing that the concept sets out the range of what qualifies as a health matter (well-being and social welfare in addition to the absence of disease) and guides researchers in their applied work. The update takes the advice of the burgeoning life course literature and directs population health scholars to fully embrace the notion of promoting health over the life course by defining health *as* well-being over the entire life course. We may often need to measure health and disease at a single point in time, as if it were a static state or a short-term process. But I insist that we should always keep in mind that, various measurement challenges aside, health is a trajectory that extends over the entire lifespan, developing through dynamic interaction with one's social context. As seen above, it is a conception that has been operationalized in venues such as the 2013 update to cholesterol management guidelines (basing treatment decisions on likelihood of net harm in a patient's foreseeable future) (Finkel and Duffy 2015; Stone et al. 2014), and the 2015 UN-WHO Every Woman, Every Child program, which links health promotion of women and children in a holistic life course attempt to disrupt well-being harms spread across the life cycle (Every Woman Every Child 2015).

The inclusiveness and flexibility of the WHO definition strike a balance between pluralism and specificity. It sets up a range of domains as legitimate components of health. How can we be sure that the WHO definition of health can be used effectively and fortuitously in actual practice? Ultimately, the proof of the pudding is in the eating, so to speak. The next chapter will explore and defend broad models of public health, which seek to address the full set of causes of benefit and harm to populations' holistic well-being, extending far outside the medical realm into areas such as economic reforms to address the health impacts of poverty. Curiously, though, such broad models of public health action have faced some of its staunchest opposition from philosophers of public health, who have been concerned about the "boundary problem" of where to draw the boundaries for the domain of public health, fearing that a lack of such boundaries would be philosophically untenable or practically disastrous. But first, this chapter will conclude with a case study of what a holistic life course perspective offers to the ongoing efforts to reduce inequitable health disparities between Aboriginal Australians and settler Australians.

Case study: addressing health disparities between Aboriginal Australians and settler Australians

Much rests on the definition of health used to develop population health research and interventions. Approximately 3 percent of Australians are Indigenous People, which includes Aboriginal Australians (90 percent of the Indigenous population), the smaller Torres Strait Islander population (6 percent), and those who identify as both (4 percent) (Australian Institute of Health and Welfare 2014: 297). Brutal colonial settlement decimated the population, in a variation on the well-known colonial tropes of land displacement, legal disempowerment, denial of suffrage, etc. The effects on the geographically diffuse population of Aboriginal Australians have been devastating—poverty, lack of access to schools, overcrowded housing, low rates of home ownership, and a multitude of other social disparities reinforcing patterns of relatively poor health in virtually every measure (Australian Institute of Health and Welfare 2015). A 2008 joint local–national government initiative committed the country to "Closing the Gap" (echoing the title of the landmark WHO social determinants of health report from the same year) (Commission on Social Determinants of Health 2008; see history in Australian Institute of Health and Welfare 2015). Focusing on Aboriginal Australians for the purpose of this case study, we can see how the evolving strategies for effecting health and well-being reforms to promote equitable treatment of Aboriginal Australians combine holistic social well-being concepts and Life Course Theory in population health promotion. Taket has explored the human rights dimensions of Aboriginal Australian health efforts, but here I am focusing on the role of health concepts (Taket 2012).

A 2015 government report reminds readers that, "[c]entral to 'Closing the Gap' is the recognition that good health is not determined solely by the presence or absence of pathogens and the failure of bodily functions," citing factors such as employment, housing conditions, breastfeeding, and various other factors (Australian Institute of Health and Welfare 2015: 3). The report goes on to explain that this multitude of social determinants indicates that a life course approach to interventions is wisest:

> the earlier in a person's life that health and welfare interventions occur, the better the outcomes for that person later in life ... possibilities for closing the gap are much greater when there is a focus on families, and on maternal and childhood health and welfare, including living conditions.
>
> (Australian Institute of Health and Welfare 2015: 3)

This is partly illustrated by Figure 3.1, which shows that diabetes rates and risks disproportionately afflict Indigenous Australians even in young adulthood, quickly building from there to devastatingly high rates in middle age and beyond.

The deep social roots of these health disparities in Australia call for models of measurement and analysis that are suited to detecting colonialism's socially embedded causes of health harm and detecting socially embedded well-being effects.

The national government's current strategy for Aboriginal health is committed to the principle: "There is a full and ongoing participation by Aboriginal and Torres Strait Islander people and organisations in all levels of decision-making affecting their health needs" (Australian Government 2013). The government of Australia has explicitly adopted a commitment to a life course approach to the health of Indigenous Australians: "A life course approach is necessary in order to address the inter-generational mechanisms that impact on health inequalities" (Australian Government 2013: 27; see also Government of

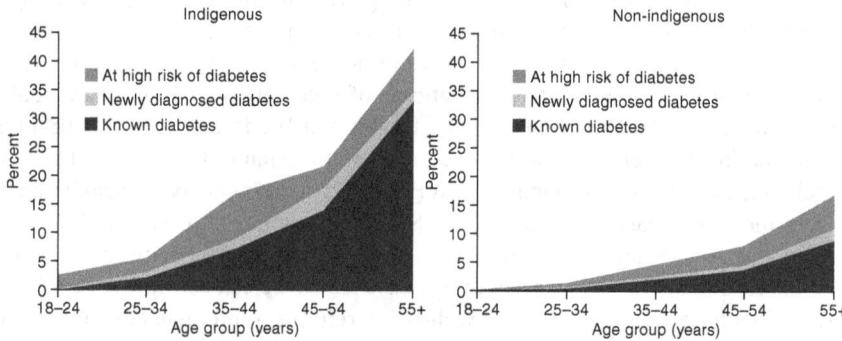

Figure 3.1 Age-specific prevalence rates of diabetes and those at high risk among people aged 18 and over, by indigenous status, 2012–2013.

Source: Australian Institute of Health and Welfare 2015: 93.

Western Australia Department of Health 2015: 10), though these commitments come with challenges. For example, a national-level health promotion framework for the years 2013–2023, and a state-level framework for the years 2015–2030 (among other such efforts) are both ambitiously long-term and yet also too short term to be capable of showing a full range of life course effects. Take, for example, efforts to address disproportionate rates of chronic disease and low birth weight. Inadequately managed chronic diseases such as diabetes (especially if undetected and unaddressed during prenatal care) are a cause of low birth weight (Government of Western Australia Department of Health 2015). Low birth weight is, in turn, a cause of diabetes in adulthood (Harder et al. 2007). But disrupting this cycle at one or multiple points in the life cycle will only yield limited measurable impacts until the adult health of yet-to-be-born children can be assessed, though other goals, such as the recruitment and retention of a larger Aboriginal health workforce (expanding capacity for culturally appropriate care), can be achieved and measured in shorter timeframes (Government of Western Australia Department of Health 2015).

Since health is inseparable from social context—in my view and in the view adopted by the previously cited efforts in Australia—population health promotion cannot proceed effectively without carefully identifying the social dynamics at play. As Jayasinghe frames it, the nuances of colonialism and racism make Aboriginal Australians "a world apart from the lives of civil servants in Whitehall" (see Chapter 2 on the groundbreaking Whitehall Study). We cannot simply assume that whatever does or does not work for addressing the classist health disparities Marmot et al. first identified in the UK, will similarly work in Australia (Jayasinghe 2011: 2; Marmot et al. 1984). Australia is working to overcome that challenge of context-specific social dynamics of well-being by first accepting that dependence and then crafting interventions that leverage those powerful social contexts to solve health problems.

A vital component of the Australian response has been to make culture and local social knowledge central, as outlined in the 2013 national-level report (Australian Government 2013) and further developed by a state-level report:

- *Ethical commitments*: "cultural security" is a "guiding principle" (Government of Western Australia Department of Health 2015: 1).
- *Leadership*: "The Framework has been developed for Aboriginal people by Aboriginal people" (Government of Western Australia Department of Health 2015: 3).
- *Research Methods*: "Aboriginal community control and engagement" (Government of Western Australia Department of Health 2015: 1).
- *Targets for interventions*: Another government report: "Connection to land, spirituality and ancestry, kinship networks, and cultural continuity are commonly identified by Aboriginal people as important health-protecting factors. These are said to serve as sources of resilience and as a unique reservoir of strength and recovery when faced with adversity" (Zubrick et al. 2014: 104).

- *Goals*: "Building community capacity" and "A strong, skilled and growing Aboriginal health workforce" (Government of Western Australia Department of Health 2015: 1).

Western Australia literally puts "culture" at the center of the diagram for its framework for health promotion of the Aboriginal population of the state. This reflects an ethical commitment to cultural "integrity" and "security" and a pragmatic recognition that its efforts to promote health and well-being will fail if they are not carefully tailored to the cultural context (Government of Western Australia Department of Health 2015).

This case study has particular philosophical import because it has been previously presented as an exception that illustrates the weakness of WHO's concept of health. Boddington and Räisänen argue that an Aboriginal Australian definition of health is incompatible with the WHO definition (Boddington and Räisänen 2009):

> Health is defined not only as physical, mental, and social but also as cultural. And several aspects are incorporated into the definition of health, notably reference to the whole of the life course, self-determination, community and culture as well as dignity and justice.
>
> (Boddington and Räisänen 2009: 57)

While I agree with most of their other aims and arguments, I argue Boddington and Räisänen misinterpret WHO's very inclusive definition of health when they take it to be exclusive of anything not expressly mentioned therein. Their critique of the concept for being too narrow makes a similar misstep, as the previously discussed critiques, that it is too broad (Daniels 2006; Hausman 2015). It is a strained interpretation of "state of complete physical, mental and social well-being and not merely the absence of disease or infirmity" to read this as exclusive of cultural variation. In fact, one of the benefits of incorporating Life Course Theory into the WHO holistic health concept is that it links new Western biomedical knowledge with the older knowledge of Aboriginal Australians.

Participatory and locally appropriate processes are absolutely vital to population health promotion for ethical reasons, but it is easy to forget that this is also because the flow of knowledge should flow in both directions during interactions between population health practitioners and the populations being served. The case of the dynamics of settler–indigenous health policies in Australia is particularly illuminating since Boddington and Räisänen show how the Aboriginal Australian concept of health includes a "temporal holism" that Australian policymakers recognized for its connection to a "lifecourse approach" (Boddington and Räisänen 2009: 61). While "temporal holism" is deeply embedded in Aboriginal culture, mainstream epidemiology only started to incorporate its parallel concept of life course health in the 1990s (Shanahan et al. 2016).

Aboriginal Australians were forced to wait for non-Aboriginal health scientists to catch up theoretically and gradually prepare themselves to accept an understanding of health causation and metaphysics that had long been part of the overarching Aboriginal Australian knowledge system. And that is finally paying off in venues such as the 2015–2030 health promotion framework for Western Australia (Government of Western Australia Department of Health 2015). This chapter's case study and the previous chapter's case study on Standing Rock Sioux health both illustrate how and why health promotion in indigenous populations requires careful implementation of lessons from population health science, and how population health science requires implementation of lessons from Indigenous populations.

Notes

1 Life course theory is distinct from evolutionary biology's "life history theory," which Griffiths and Matthewson have used to help resolve objections about whether a naturalistic concept of health can properly account for normal bodily changes during aging (Griffiths and Matthewson 2016).
2 It is possible to reconcile a naturalistic more or less Biostatistical concept of disease with an acceptance of a positive concept of health; Williams does this by splitting disease and health such that he gives a disease account similar to Boorse's but concludes with a qualified endorsement of the WHO concept of health: "WHO overstates what is needed for health," but, "the denial that health is merely the absence of disease is surely correct" (Williams 2007).

Works cited

Arah, O. A. (2009) On the relationship between individual and population health. *Medicine, Health Care and Philosophy* 12, 235–244.

Australian Government. (2013) National Aboriginal and Torres Strait Islander Health Plan. Canberra: Commonwealth of Australia.

Australian Institute of Health and Welfare. (2014) Australia's health 2014. www.aihw.gov.au/publication-detail/?id=60129547205: Australian Institute of Health and Welfare.

Australian Institute of Health and Welfare. (2015) The health and welfare of Australia's Aboriginal and Torres Strait Islander peoples 2015. www.aihw.gov.au/WorkArea/DownloadAsset.aspx?id=60129551281: Australian Institute of Health and Welfare.

Backholer, K., Beauchamp, A., Ball, K., et al. (2014) A framework for evaluating the impact of obesity prevention strategies on socioeconomic inequalities in weight. *American Journal of Public Health* 104, e43-e50.

Bell, K. (2017) *Health and Other Unassailable Values: Reconfigurations of Health, Evidence and Ethics*. London: Routledge.

Bickenbach, J. (2015) WHO's Definition of Health: Philosophical Analysis. In: Schramme, T. and Edwards, S. (eds) *Handbook of the Philosophy of Medicine*. Dordrecht: Springer Netherlands, 1–14.

Boddington, P. and Räisänen, U. (2009) Theoretical and practical issues in the definition of health: Insights from Aboriginal Australia. *Journal of Medicine and Philosophy* 34, 49–67.

Boorse, C. (1977) Health as a theoretical concept. *Philosophy of Science* 44, 542–573.

Boorse, C. (2014) A second rebuttal on health. *Journal of Medicine and Philosophy* 39, 683–724.

Callahan, D. (1973) The WHO definition of "health." *The Hastings Center Report* 1, 77–87.

Carel, H. and Cooper, R. (2014) *Health, Illness and Disease: Philosophical Essays*. New York: Routledge.

Coggon, J. (2012) *What Makes Health Public? A Critical Evaluation of Moral, Legal, and Political Claims in Public Health*. New York: Cambridge University Press.

Commission on Social Determinants of Health. (2008) Closing the Gap in a Generation: Health Equity Through Action on the Social Determinants of Health. Geneva: World Health Organization.

Corbin, J. and Strauss, A. (1988) *Unending Work and Care: Managing Chronic Illness at Home*. San Francisco, CA: Jossey-Bass.

Daniels, N. (2006) Equity and population health: Toward a broader bioethics agenda. *Hastings Center Report* 36, 22–35.

Edington, D. W., Schultz, A. B. and Pitts, J. S. (2016) The Future of Population Health at the Workplace: Trends, Technology, and the Role of Mind-Body and Behavioral Sciences In: Nash, D. B., Fabius, R. J., Skoufalos, A., et al. (eds) *Population Health: Creating a Culture of Wellness*. Burlington, MA: Jones & Bartlett Learning.

Elder, G. H., Kirkpatrick Johnson, M. and Crosnoe, R. (2003) The Emergence and Development of Life Course Theory. In: Mortimer, J. T. and Shanahan, M. J. (eds) *Handbook of the Life Course*. New York: Kluwer Academic, 3–19.

Evans, R. G. and Stoddart, G. L. (1990) Producing health, consuming health care. *Social Science and Medicine* 31, 1347–1363.

Every Woman Every Child. (2015) The global strategy for women's, children's and adolescents' health. United Nations.

Finkel, J. B. and Duffy, D. (2015) 2013 ACC/AHA cholesterol treatment guideline: Paradigm shifts in managing atherosclerotic cardiovascular disease risk. *Trends in Cardiovascular Medicine* 25, 340–347.

Fuller, J. (2017) What are chronic diseases? *Synthese*, 1–24.

GBD 2015 Mortality and Causes of Death Collaborators. (2016) Global, regional, and national life expectancy, all-cause mortality, and cause-specific mortality for 249 causes of death, 1980–2015: A systematic analysis for the Global Burden of Disease Study 2015. *The Lancet* 388, 1459–1544.

Giroux, É. (2015) Epidemiology and the bio-statistical theory of disease: A challenging perspective. *Theoretical Medicine and Bioethics* 36, 175–195.

Goff, D. C., Lloyd-Jones, D. M., Bennett, G., et al. (2013) 2013 ACC/AHA guideline on the assessment of cardiovascular risk. *Circulation* 63, 2935–2959.

Government of Western Australia Department of Health. (2015) WA Aboriginal Health and Wellbeing Framework 2015–2030. http://ww2.health.wa.gov.au/Improving-WA-Health/About-Aboriginal-Health/WA-Aboriginal-Health-and-Wellbeing-Framework-2015-2030: Department of Health.

Griffiths, P. E. and Matthewson, J. (2016) Evolution, dysfunction, and disease: A reappraisal. *The British Journal for the Philosophy of Science*. Available at: https://doi.org/10.1093/bjps/axw021.

Harder, T., Rodekamp, E., Schellong, K., et al. (2007) Birth weight and subsequent risk of type 2 diabetes: A meta-analysis. *American Journal of Epidemiology* 165, 849–857.

Hausman, D. M. (2015) *Valuing Health: Well-Being, Freedom and Suffering*. New York: Oxford University Press.

Humber, J. M. and Almeder, R. F. (2010) *What Is Disease?* Totowa, NJ: Humana Press.

International Conference on Population and Development. (1994) Report of the International Conference on Population and Development. New York: United Nations.

Irwin, A. and Scali, E. (2007) Action on the social determinants of health: A historical perspective. *Global Public Health* 2, 235–256.

Jayasinghe, S. (2011) Conceptualising population health: From mechanistic thinking to complexity science. *Emerging Themes in Epidemiology* 8, 2.

Keyes, K. M. and Galea, S. (2016) *Population Health Science*. New York: Oxford University Press.

Kindig, D. and Stoddart, G. (2003) What is population health? *American Journal of Public Health* 93, 380–383.

Kindig, D. A. (2007) Understanding population health terminology. *Milbank Quarterly* 85, 139–161.

Krueger, J. (2015) Theoretical health and medical practice. *Philosophy of Science* 82, 491–508.

Kukla, R. (2010) The ethics and cultural politics of reproductive risk warnings: A case study of California's Proposition 65. *Health, Risk & Society* 12, 323–334.

Labonté, R. (1995) Population health and health promotion: What do they have to say to each other? *Canadian Journal of Public Health* 86, 165–168.

Lemoine, M. (2013) Defining disease beyond conceptual analysis: An analysis of conceptual analysis in philosophy of medicine. *Theoretical Medicine and Bioethics* 34, 309–325.

Marmot, M. G., Shipley, M. J. and Rose, G. (1984) Inequalities in death—specific explanations of a general pattern? *The Lancet* 323, 1003–1006.

May, T., Byonanebye, J. and Meurer, J. (2017) The ethics of population health management: Collapsing the traditional boundary between patient care and public health. *Population Health Management* 20, 167–169.

Metzl, J. and Kirkland, A. (2010) *Against Health: How Health Became the New Morality*. New York: New York University Press.

Morales-Asencio, J. M., Martin-Santos, F. J., Kaknani, S., et al. (2016) Living with chronicity and complexity: Lessons for redesigning case management from patients' life stories: A qualitative study. *Journal of Evaluation in Clinical Practice* 22, 122–132.

Nordenfelt, L. (2016) A Defence of a Holistic Concept of Health. In: Giroux, É. (ed.) *Naturalism in the Philosophy of Health: Issues and Implications.* Cham: Springer International Publishing, 209–225.

Nussbaum, M. C. (2011) *Creating Capabilities: The Human Development Approach.* Cambridge: Belknap Press.

Ohri-Vachaspati, P., Isgor, Z., Rimkus, L., et al. (2015) Child-directed marketing inside and on the exterior of fast-food restaurants. *American Journal of Preventive Medicine* 48, 22–30.

Powers, M. and Faden, R. R. (2006) *Social Justice: The Moral Foundations of Public Health and Health Policy*. New York: Oxford University Press.

Ruger, J. P. (2010) *Health and Social Justice*. Oxford: Oxford University Press.

Schwartz, P. H. (2014) Reframing the disease debate and defending the biostatistical theory. *Journal of Medicine and Philosophy* 39, 572–589.

Sen, A. (2004) Health Achievement and Equity: External and Internal Perspectives. In: Anand, S., Peter, F. and Sen, A. (eds) *Public Health, Ethics, and Equity.* Oxford: Oxford University Press, 263–268.

Sen, A. (2005) Human rights and capabilities. *Journal of Human Development* 6, 151–166.

Shanahan, M. J., Mortimer, J. T. and Johnson, M. K. (2016) Introduction: Life Course Studies—Trends, Challenges, and Future Directions. In: Shanahan, M. J., Mortimer, J. T. and Johnson, M. K. (eds) *Handbook of the Life Course*. New York: Springer, 1–23.

Smart, B. (2014) On the classification of diseases. *Theoretical Medicine and Bioethics* 35, 251–269.

Stone, N. J., Robinson, J. G., Lichtenstein, A. H., et al. (2014) 2013 ACC/AHA guideline on the treatment of blood cholesterol to reduce atherosclerotic cardiovascular risk in adults. *Journal of the American College of Cardiology* 63, 2889–2934.

Taket, A. (2012) *Health Equity, Social Justice and Human Rights*. Abingdon: Routledge.

Venkatapuram, S. (2011) *Health Justice: An Argument from the Capabilities Approach*. Malden, MA: Polity Press.

Williams, N. E. (2007) The factory model of disease. *The Monist* 90, 555–584.

World Health Organization. (1946) Official Records of the World Health Organization. *International Health Conference*. New York: United Nations.

World Health Organization. (2014) Twelfth General Programme of Work 2014–2019: Not merely the absence of disease. Geneva: World Health Organization.

World Health Organization Regional Committee for Europe. (2016) Action plan for sexual and reproductive health: Towards achieving the 2030 Agenda for Sustainable Development in Europe—leaving no one behind. Copenhagen: World Health Organization.

Young, T. K. (2005) *Population Health: Concepts and Methods*. New York: Oxford University Press.

Zubrick, S. R., Shepherd, C. C. J., Dudgeon, P., et al. (2014) Social Determinants of Social and Emotional Wellbeing. In: Dudgeon, P., Milroy, H. and Walker, R. (eds) *Working Together: Aboriginal and Torres Strait Islander Mental Health and Wellbeing Principles and Practice*. www.mhcc.org.au/media/80434/working-together-aboriginal-and-wellbeing-2014.pdf, 93–112.

Part II

Which causes and effects matter most in population health?

4 Expanding the boundaries of population health

Introduction: health as a life course of complete well-being in social context calls for a broad health promotion mandate

In the 2010s it has become a truism that public/population health must adopt a broad model; that is, health promotion efforts need to use a variety of means to target the full array of social and environmental determinants of health. Relying on governmental mandates to target a shifting subset of behavioral and genetic determinants is far from adequate. We must attend to the health implications of any and all policies, from commercial/residential zoning laws (which control the relative neighborhood availability of alcohol, fast food, groceries, etc.; Rudolph et al. 2013), to food advertising practices (which shape children's food preferences; Ohri-Vachaspati et al. 2015), to the ease of forming labor unions (which affect workplace safety and bargaining for a living wage; Hagedorn et al. 2016). This embrace of a broad model of health promotion, beyond government-led or healthcare-centered efforts, is well established.

Despite broad models' popularity among population health practitioners, such wide-scope efforts have been staunchly opposed by many philosophers of public health, who maintain that there is a grave "boundary problem" that must be attended to—they contend that we must set careful limits on what qualifies as a (public) health matter. As I have previously argued (Valles 2016), this leaves an unsettlingly wide gap between practitioners of public health and philosophers of public health. The gap is perhaps most starkly illustrated by the juxtaposition of the official position of the American Public Health Association (APHA) and the position taken by Mark Rothstein, the associate editor for the ethics section of the APHA's journal, *American Journal of Public Health*. The APHA is a staunch advocate of broad public health (e.g., it partnered with the Public Health Institute to write a guidebook to help policymakers implement Health in All Policies) (Rudolph et al. 2013). And the APHA joined 57 other medical and public health organizations in pleading for the US to expand its collection of data on gun violence and its implementation of gun restrictions (American Pediatric Association et al. 2016). Meanwhile, Rothstein has been a leading opponent of broad models of public health, and rejects the inclusion of crime and other social ills as part of "the public health agenda"—since this would render "public health ... so broad as to be meaning-less" (Rothstein 2009: 87).

Asserting the existence of a "boundary problem" puts philosophers out of step with the public/population health practitioners they study. This divide calls out for attention to not only the views of each side, but also to what could be responsible for the distance between the two camps. I argue below that philo-sophers' concerns of a boundary problem largely stem from misunderstandings of what population health models are and what effects they have had. It is a long-standing concern among philosophers of medicine that broad concepts of health, such as the WHO definition of health, run the risk of "turn[ing] all prob-lems of 'social well-being' over to the medical professional" (Callahan 1973: 82). Ceding all matters of social welfare to medical professionals would indeed be a horrible idea. As the next section will argue, adopting a broad-scoped vision of health and of health promotion activities does not commit population health science to ceding social welfare to medical professionals. Quite the opposite—population health science is built atop the hard-learned lesson that health is a sprawling thing that results from many domains of social life outside of medicine/healthcare and requiring interventions outside the healthcare sector. A broad model of population health under a population health science philosophy refuses to be constrained by the boundary problem, but it does *not* march us toward a future where health experts wield ever more social power. Population health sci-ence's models of action are founded on humble acceptance of the fact that health experts cannot dictate effective health policies from on high. "Health is created and lived by people within the settings of their everyday life (World Health Organization 1986b)," which requires a correspondingly wide range of know-ledge and actors working together to create "a culture of health (Nash et al. 2016; Gottlieb et al. 2016)" through "engagement and collaboration across sectors (World Health Organization 2015: 3)."

Continuing from Chapter 3: "health issues" ≠ "healthcare issues"

Onyebuchi Arah, whose work was featured in Chapter 3, helps to illuminate the ways that population health-thinking serves to challenge philosophers' ingrained intuitions (Arah 2009). That chapter elaborated on Arah's demonstration that the presumptive firm boundary between individual health and population health breaks down when we adopt a life course population health perspective; indi-vidual health and population health dynamically and mutually affect each other over the gradual passage of time (Arah 2009). He also challenges the assumption that a health-as-well-being concept (such as the WHO definition or my variation on it, using his life course insights) proves its own absurdity by having health grow to be (more or less) coextensive with total well-being. This is connected to his rebuttal against criticisms of health-as-well-being concepts (e.g., the one pro-posed by WHO, and which I elaborated on), saying they are "refreshingly bold" for so seriously responding to the lesson that health affects, and is affected by, virtually every aspect of human life (Arah 2009). After all, the daunting lesson of the twentieth century, as traced in Chapter 2, is that health is entirely enmeshed in human social life. I share his suspicion that philosophers' resistance to broad concepts of health is largely rooted in a "fear of medicalization" (Arah 2009: 241). That is, if health's boundaries expand to include all human well-being then the fear is that surely healthcare would grow along with it. We have ample reason to fear an unguided expansion of healthcare's domain; it would serve to encourage the hegemony of a healthcare industry always looking to find, or create, a new problem to solve with its costly goods and services (González-Moreno et al. 2015), among innumerable other abuses of power (Metzl and Kirkland 2010; Bell 2017).

The fears that healthcare's authority will grow along with an expansion of the health concept, though, are misguided. They rely on adopting an assumption that population health was founded to reject: the assumption that the healthcare sector is the rightful leader of health promotion efforts. Over four decades ago, the Lalonde Report surmised that there was already compelling theoretical and empirical evidence to the contrary (Lalonde 1974). As shown in Chapter 2, a population's health is attributable to all manner of social features totally outside of healthcare. As Arah puts it, "not every health need would become a healthcare need. In this sense, health need subsumes healthcare need, not the other way around" (Arah 2009: 241). In a related point, Sholl warns against conflating concerns over medicalization with concerns over pathologization—the act of recognizing that some biological process or experience is pathological does not automatically mean one is simultaneously recognizing medicine as the proper means of addressing it—for example, one can recognize an ailment as a distinct pathology that should be left to "run its course" (Sholl 2017: 272).

Arah's point about philosophers conflating health and healthcare, helps to make sense of the boundary problem. While the boundary problem is most actively discussed in the public health ethics literature, it is described quite lucidly in *Philosophy of Epidemiology*, Alex Broadbent's text on epistemology/ evidence, metaphysics and philosophy of science in epidemiology. Broadbent sees that epidemiologists' research often serves to put pressure on healthcare policy by making a *prima facie* case for why it would make sense to expand the purview of medicine—he uses the example of research linking internet use and suicide, which raises questions about medical professionals' role(s) in addressing this empirical finding (Broadbent 2013). The fear is that when we find some X causally benefits or harms health, we then use that as a rationale for expanding the domain of medical professionals to then include X. Should we now give medical experts new power over internet regulation? Does every new discovery of the health effects of a social cause mean we should cede some additional authority over it to medical experts? This is the boundary problem.

"Boundary problem" problems

Concerns about the boundary problem are not baseless. Broadbent shows the logical fallacy of those who would argue: doctors are responsible for contending with many "causes of ill health" and therefore anything known to be a cause of ill health will automatically be a doctor's concern. Logically, it does not follow. He offers the example of a hypothetical impending meteor strike, using it to build up a counterargument against those who would expand the domain of medicine whenever a new health threat emerges. In doing so, he explicitly targets Michael Marmot, the leader of the pivotal Whitehall Study of social determinants of health and lead author of the landmark WHO report on that topic (Commission on Social Determinants of Health 2008), discussed in Chapter 2. Broadbent allows that a "medical response" to the hypothetical meteor strike would be appropriate:

> if such a strike were predicted or occurred unpredicted; but it is surely not the job of the medical profession to anticipate it. If not, then Michael Marmot's argument that social inequality is a concern of the physician's because it causes ill health (Marmot 2006b) is fallacious.
>
> (Broadbent 2013: 147)

Medical professionals are indeed limited in their respective scientific expertise. Epidemiologists would be fools to pretend they have the astronomical skills to predict a meteorite hitting the earth. Broadbent elaborates that the same goes for normative matters; epidemiologists have roles to play in public debate but need to stay in their lane—so to speak—when it comes to ethical matters.

> Epidemiologists can tell us what the benefits and costs of a smoke-free or a stair-free society would be for population health; but it is not their job to decide whether the benefits are worth the costs.
>
> (Broadbent 2013: 148)

It might seem rather unobjectionable to want epidemiologists and other medical professionals to stay within strict professional boundaries, but such boundaries lose their luster when examined more closely.

Broadbent's critique helps to illuminate a common, but mistaken, philosophical assumption—the idea that we can split apart the descriptive and normative aspects of population health science in the first place. Katikireddi and I begin a 2015 paper arguing for the coupled analysis of ethical and evidentiary aspects of public health (recognizing that ethical and evidentiary aspects of science are tied together), by noting that the scientific practices aim at the ethical goal of health equity: "it is widely accepted that a fundamental purpose of public health is ameliorating unacceptable health inequalities or health disparities" (Katikireddi and Valles 2015: e36). As defined in the contemporary population health textbook, population health "seeks to promote ... effective, equitable, ethical, and accessible care" (Sidorov and Romney 2016: 21); ethical judgments and the pursuit of ethical objectives are core components of population health science practice (Keyes and Galea 2016a), as further elaborated in the section below on "epistemic risk." In the case of Marmot and his WHO Commission, the team pointedly declares on the back cover of its report: "reducing health inequities is, for the Commission on Social Determinants of Health, an ethical imperative. Social injustice is killing people on a grand scale" (Commission on Social Determinants of Health 2008). They justify their broad mandate from this empirical fact and the ethical condemnation of that fact. To reiterate lessons from Chapter 2, the public health community's discovery of health's empirical roots in social life, including blatant social injustices, led to the community adopting the ethical task of remedying the injustices; this ethical goal then led to the development of new methods for addressing health harms deeply rooted in social life. The ethics of population health science cannot be bracketed off from the rest of the science.

It is not only impossible to extract the ethical elements of population health science from the other components, but the interdisciplinary natures of both public health and population health can lead to confusion about what is or is not proper behavior for the diverse experts within these endeavors. Broadbent's language shifts between referring to "the medical profession," "physicians," and "epidemiologists" in his discussion of the boundary problem—seemingly to say that all of these experts need to restrict their professional efforts (Broadbent 2013: 147–148). But, as Arah counsels, we must not conflate the domain of *health* needs/solutions with the domain of *healthcare* needs/solutions (Arah 2009). We should absolutely knock down the boundaries that obstruct broad population health promotion, allowing us to address social determinants of health such as inequitable tax burdens on the poor, but that does not mean we should let the *healthcare* sector plant its flag and claim ultimate authority over economic policy. Health and healthcare are distinct; epidemiological research and clinical medicine are distinct.

It is an entirely separate question *who* in the population health interdisciplinary community should respond to a given problem—such as Broadbent's example of internet use and suicide—and how. A population health response could very well include no clinical healthcare personnel at all. In the case of internet use, it may end up being best to respond though a program of: monitoring by epidemiologists; qualitative investigation by sociologists and anthropologists; and preventive public education efforts in schools, religious institutions, and other community organizations. I have no objection to limiting the professional domain or behavior of individual types of experts within interdisciplinary and intersectoral population health science, while still maintaining that population health science, *as a whole*, must engage with all aspects of the causes and effects of health in human populations.

Political theory and population health

As Harris et al. aptly summarize in their contrasting of population health from public health, "population health uses public health tools and techniques to identify and intervene at the community level," including "tackling large-scale social, economic, and environmental issues" (Harris et al. 2016: 40). By contrast, "public health is generally seen as a tool of state and federal government exercising its sovereign and constitutionally authorized police power" (Harris et al. 2016: 40). Using this latter understanding of public health allows one to analyze the government–individual conflicts in cases such as state-imposed quarantines, but applying this same theoretical lens brings little clarity to cases of population health promotion *outside* of government control. At worst, advocates of this theoretical lens try to block population health promotion that does not conform to this narrow model of public health as state action.

The staunchest philosophical opposition to a broad mandate for population/ public health is rooted in the classical liberal theory of philosophy. This work in political philosophy posits and investigates the push and pull between individual liberty vs. state interests. This framing of public health as tension between individual and government leads to an ethical approach, which has been well articulated by Rothstein (2002, 2009):

> "Government intervention as public health" involves public officials taking appropriate measures pursuant to specific legal authority, after balancing private rights and public interests, to protect the health of the public.
>
> (Rothstein 2002: 146)

Rothstein is dismayed by the idea of a population health science model—a model that challenges this duality by denying that government (or its agents) is necessarily one of the two parties.

> The "population health as public health" approach is thus ill-defined, with diverse actors pursuing widely divergent strategies to deal with the same health problems, tackling health problems of varying severity, and often pursuing their own agendas with little coordination or accountability.
>
> (Rothstein 2002: 146)

He further argues that it is "ill-advised," to adopt a broad population health approach. The mixing of "government with non-government initiatives" muddies the legal/moral authority being invoked (Rothstein 2002: 146). The main practical consequence of his rejection "is simply that resolution of underlying socioeconomic and political problems is beyond the domain of public health" (Rothstein 2009: 86).

Rothstein's liberal political theory priorities are rooted in legitimate worries about the need to limit the power of government, much like the previously discussed "boundary problem" is rooted in legitimate worries about the need to limit the power of healthcare and various health professions. Population health science is in no way theoretically opposed to such concerns. In fact, the discovery that even mundane government policies (e.g., sidewalk design in urban planning) can have serious health impacts (e.g., cardiovascular health effects of physical exercise) gives population health science additional motivation to scrutinize government action (Rudolph et al. 2013).

Holland, in his prominent contemporary public health ethics text, conveys his thought processes in rejecting a broad model of public health. Early in the text he ponders whether he ought to write a book that is "conceptually, politically and geographically ambitious, and advocate[s] global change," but he decides against (Holland 2015: 5), also doubting he will convince "highly politicized readers" to similarly embrace this narrower view of public health and public health ethics. He goes so far as to dismiss such scholars as not scholars at all—a "reader" advocating for such a program is a "reformer, as opposed to a scholar" (Holland 2015: 6). If ambitious ethical goals and a recognition of the ethical need for political reform fall outside his conception of mainstream public health ethics then that speaks volumes about just how far Public Health Ethics work can drift from the real world ethical challenges of public health.

In his political theory-framing of public health ethics, Hausman's book on health measurement philosophy draws a dichotomy between "private" vs. "public" values; each person's health makes valuable contributions to the pursuit of their individual interests (e.g., my physical fitness is valuable to my personal parenting goal of keeping pace with my daughter's active lifestyle), and certain value to the public's interests (e.g., my variety of physical fitness conforms to what US health policy considers appropriate for a healthy person who needs relatively few resources) (Hausman 2015: 157). However, Hausman sees all public interests flowing through the state; a society has interests in certain aspects of its members' health and promotes its interests through health policies via the state as "their agent," with the state sometimes "delegating details" of those policies "to individuals and other institutions" (Hausman 2015: 154). This hews closely to an individual vs. state dichotomy of public health deliberations.

The works of Rothstein, Holland, and Hausman all offer prominent examples of how individual vs. state liberalist philosophy serves to funnel debates over proper public health action into a model of public health as an expression of government authority. This preemptively shuts out engagement with population health science, since population health science denies this dichotomy and instead demands collaboration between sectors (see Chapter 8). The science is predicated on the need to let the particularities of the population health issue dictate which sectors of society are involved, and how. The state does not automatically have pride of place in population health efforts. Each person's health is both benefitted and harmed by a dizzying constellation of causes over the course of a social life. Few of those causes are directly managed by the state. In the US, a survey of hospitals indicates those (usually non-governmental) institutions are eager advocates of a shift toward "population health" models for serving their communities; it is their prerogative to follow through even if the government decides to reject such models (Health Research & Educational Trust 2015).

The literature on population health science and governance is quite open about the fact that the state is actually incapable of dictating a sufficient set of top-down health promotion policies (McQueen et al. 2012b). Instead, the state can accept a role as facilitator or coordinator of intersectoral collaborations that are mutually agreeable to all actors; it is "imperative to facilitate governance practices that enable improved work across sectors in government, the non-government sector, academic institutions and the private sector, at all territorial levels" (McQueen et al. 2012b: ix). Population health interventions are only sometimes manifestations of state power (whether direct or indirect), so it is ineffectual to critique it under the model of a citizenry setting limits on the government via collective will and consent to be governed. I am not the first philosopher to push back against narrow public health models, though: I adopt the "broad" vs. "narrow" phrasing favored by Daniel Goldberg in his rebuttal to Rothstein's conception of public health as necessarily a highly constrained exercise of state authority (Goldberg 2009).

Goldberg offers compelling public health ethics rebuttals to "boundary problem objections," rooted in Bruce Link and Jo Phelan's groundbreaking "fundamental causes" theory and makes some use of the Health in All Policies model (Goldberg 2014). Central to the account of health causation that will be expounded in Chapter 5, "fundamental cause" theory gives an empirically supported model for "upstream" social and environmental features of human life (e.g., wealth) as the root causes of innumerable "downstream" health effects (Link and Phelan 1995). Goldberg seeks to defuse concerns about the boundary problem as a means of defending Madison Powers and Ruth Faden's "health sufficiency model of social justice" (Goldberg 2014), a variation on the "capabilities approach" in which Powers and Faden attempt to lay out what it would mean for people to have a sufficient level of well-being, expressed as human "functionings" (not just the capability to function) across six dimensions of life: "health, personal security, reasoning, respect, attachment, and self-determination" (Powers and Faden 2006: 16).

Goldberg dispenses with the empirical claim that a broad model of health promotion through social reform is not feasible—such dismissals are contradicted by an extensive record of efforts that can and do promote health through efforts outside the narrow public health mold (Goldberg 2014). He then goes on to correct additional empirical misconceptions underlying boundary problem objections to broad social reforms as means of public health promotion. Citing empirical data that such social reforms indeed tend to be cost-effective, he offers the ethical rebuttal that even high costs or political difficulties of social justice efforts do not mean they should stop being our priorities; sometimes the right thing is also the hard thing (Goldberg 2014). But Goldberg underplays the depth and breadth of "boundary problem" concerns among philosophers, most notably the boundary problem objections voiced by Powers and Faden, whose work he seeks to defend against others' "boundary problem" objections.

An unnecessary philosophical assumption: if X becomes a public health problem then it must be primarily or exclusively a public health problem

One set of boundary problem objections rest on a flawed philosophical assumption: that defining health to include many components of total well-being would steal those dimensions of well-being away from other dimensions of human life. For example, to live healthy lives, the people in my community need to be safe from intimate partner physical violence at home and safe from violent crime in our neighborhoods. But, citing either of these as health matters makes some philosophers worry that conceiving of health this way could lead to health usurping the conceptual importance of matters such as personal safety, and usurping the social structures used to address them. Does this mean that health professionals are stealing some of the authority and responsibilities of the criminal justice system? In a word, no.

A holistic concept of human health-as-well-being is not doomed to pitting social justice endeavors against each other. Health can include all of well-being without implying that every other dimension of well-being is demoted or reduced to a component of health. The error of assuming otherwise is illustrated in Powers and Faden's explanation of why they reject WHO's positive concept of health as complete well-being. Though acknowledging, "the broad scope of public health is often interpreted, we think rightly, as the correct perspective," they worry "public health is sometimes viewed as being so expansive in its compass as to have no real core, no institutional, disciplinary, or social boundaries," because ills ranging from "terrorism" to "income inequality" to "natural disasters [have] been claimed as a public health problem" (Powers and Faden 2006: 10). This is part of their worry, that defining health as well-being automatically makes all other dimensions of well-being automatically subsidiary and inferior to health, rendering health considerations the "sole moral foundation" for justifying equitable policy solutions. For example, they cite laws that oppose "female genital mutilation" on health grounds, but insist that such practices are just as much violations of two additional dimensions of well-being:

> personal security, and self-determination. In this case, the moral foundation in justice for the policies draws upon three dimensions of well-being, none of which is reducible to the others. Each signals a separate kind of injustice produced through the mutilation.
>
> (Powers and Faden 2006: 17)

I agree with this point about the multidimensional harms of coercive female genital cutting. Though I reject the meta-philosophical assumption that recognition of the health aspects necessarily lead to the elevation of health as the "sole moral foundation" for equity. They assume that a broad WHO-style understanding of health would put personal security policies under the moral aegis of health. As Young phrases the worry, "ministries of health will then become ministries of everything!" (Young 2005: 3).

This variety of concern puzzles me, as someone who never saw why health-as-complete-well-being means various components of well-being; spiritual, emotional, security, social connectedness, etc. must exist in a non-overlapping or hierarchical relationship with health. A state of complete health includes the freedom for people to obtain ritual tattoos or piercings as befitting their religions. At the same time, spiritual well-being includes this right, too, how ever one chooses to define spiritual well-being. Where is the tension? I leave it to scholars of personal security to specify what falls within their scope of concern; whether or not they claim as security issues some of the phenomena that I would also claim as health issues, I see no reason for the (meta-philosophical) presumption that we must compete for territory like opposing armies. Powers and Faden chose a particularly inapt example, since they advocate for the multidimensionality of well-being, while their own example falls into the trap of representing "female genital mutilation" as a single type of harm that necessarily violates three forms of well-being. By contrast, scholars specializing in the practices and ethics of Africa's "female genital surgeries" warn that rhetoric around "female genital mutilation" grossly oversimplifies the diversity of the relevant practices, cultural significances, and ethical considerations (The Public Policy Advisory Network on Female Genital Surgeries in Africa 2012). Sensitivity to the *multidimensionality* of human well-being first requires sensitivity to the *diversity* of human well-being. As a Jew, male genital cutting has spiritual significance to me and to my family, in addition to its medical significance, whereas male genital cutting has no bearing on the spiritual well-being of most of my neighbors. The boundaries of what qualifies as a health well-being matter, as a spiritual well-being matter, as a personal security well-being matter, etc. will vary by context, and the boundaries of each will often overlap; none of these features are inherently problematic.

Consider the case of gun violence, a prime example of a threat to personal security. We gain much from recognizing gun violence as a personal security problem *and* as a component of health. Gun violence is directly impactful on health (bullets are well known for their health effects on human bodies). And if personal security is largely a constituent part of health then it directs us to consider the entirety of policing, criminal justice, the private security industry, and all other security matters as health matters. Take, for example, the profusion of gated communities and personal firearms among White South Africans, which have partly replaced *de jure* Apartheid segregation with a de facto means of perpetuating segregation and unconscionable social inequities (Scheper-Hughes 2014). Matters of health and security (including gun ownership) overlap quite a lot. Meanwhile, many wealthy nations have disproportionately high rates of incarceration for Indigenous populations, a fact that has contributed to health disparities (King et al. 2009). More generally, personal security and health are bound together by the fact that exposure to violence and to perceptions of insecurity directly and indirectly induce physiological stresses (Kirk and Hardy 2014).

Even if all or nearly all of "personal security" (Powers and Faden 2006) impacts social well-being and hence health under the definition I support, "personal security" can still retain a distinct conceptual status and distinct practical status. Criminal justice theory and criminal justice practice remain vital. Curiously, despite their aforementioned concerns about granting a wide compass to health, Powers and Faden in other places don't seem to see overlap between dimensions of well-being as a problem. "The only claim of distinctiveness for the dimensions of well-being on our list is whether each captures a morally salient aspect of human flourishing that is not reducible to the others" (Powers and Faden 2006: 21). In this light, perhaps the motivating discomfort comes from the nature of the overlap between health and dimensions such as personal security, such that more or less all of personal security is conceptually and practically part of health, while health also includes much more than personal security.

Venkatapuram tries to resolve such overlap disputes (see also Hausman 2015) by classifying health as "meta-capability," though this solution reinforces fears that health matters will attempt to lord over all other considerations of well-being (Venkatapuram 2011; Schramme 2016). Meyer and Schwartz warn against the "public healthification of social problems," which could lead to the entire "discourse" of poverty being taken over by public health, with all other considerations excluded (Meyer and Schwartz 2000). Venkatapuram offers a viable solution to boundary disputes by treating health as a meta-capability. I prefer to just let dimensions of well-being overlap on the same level, rather than resorting to a hierarchical relationship that elevates health above other dimensions of well-being. At the very least, I insist that overlaps between health and other dimensions of well-being need not *require* us to adopt a hierarchical relationship. Health can be expansive without being hegemonic. A component of a life of well-being—access to clean water, bonding between children and their guardians, the safety to navigate one's neighborhood, etc.—can be a component of health and no less a component of some other category of well-being (spiritual, emotional, security, or whatever categories one may choose). To reverse the argument, if someone were to define spiritual well-being to include health I would feel no threat against my broad concept of health. Chapter 2's case study of Standing Rock Sioux health illustrates a case where religious well-being, environmental/ecosystem well-being, and health well-being all conceptually coincide for the Standing Rock population context. Aspects of well-being will almost surely overlap no matter how one carves up that conceptual landscape. It is a pernicious and needless additional assumption that overlapping aspects of well-being must therefore compete.

An incorrect empirical prediction: broad conceptions of public health predictably lead to harms to the public health professions or to the populations they serve

The WHO Commission on Social Determinants of Health meticulously explains the nature and scope of the ways that mundane elements of social life have clear and powerful effects on health. Recreational options, neighborhood design, cultural attitudes toward women, transportation options, workers' access to union collective bargaining, etc. are all health matters (Commission on Social Determinants of Health 2008), just as surely as issues long accepted as health matters, such as water sanitation, pharmaceutical safety, and hospital hand-washing practices.

> Improve the conditions of daily life—the circumstances in which people are born, grow, live, work, and age. Tackle the inequitable distribution of power, money, and resources—the structural drivers of those conditions of daily life—globally, nationally, and locally.
>
> (Commission on Social Determinants of Health 2008: 43)

It took time for the public/population health community to reach the point where such assertions could be heard and accepted. In the US, after a twentieth century largely devoted to "developing bio-medical sciences," under the model that "activism is at odds with the objective disposition of science," "public health was reluctant to move beyond its own professional boundaries," even after the accumulation of disturbing data on health inequities (National Association of County & City Health Officials 2014: 7–9). The solution, according to the influential National Association of County & City Health Officials, defies the boundary problem: the title of their report on the topic is "Expanding the Boundaries" (National Association of County & City Health Officials 2014).

Goldberg points to "Health in All Policies" as a promising and increasingly popular model for population health promotion. Recognizing "Health in All Policies" as a long-standing widely adopted model is a powerful means of refuting arguments that adopting such a model would lead to bad outcomes. In fact, the model fits firmly within the overarching population health science philosophy by insisting that the model must be pursued through collaboration.

> Public health agencies and organizations will need to work with those who are best positioned to create policies and practices that promote healthy communities and environments and secure the many co-benefits that can be attained through healthy public policy.
>
> (Rudolph et al. 2013: 1)

This exhortation to work collaboratively should short-circuit some of the concerns about imperialism being the next step after expanding the boundaries of population health science.

Instead, Rothstein predicts that taking on social problems as public health problems is unpromising and perhaps will even be counterproductive:

> war, famine, crime, poverty, unemployment, income inequality, environmental degradation, lack of economic development, human rights violations, poor education, inadequate housing, lack of natural resources and unresponsive governments. Calling these societal problems "public health" issues

does nothing to bring about their remediation and ... may actually impede their amelioration.

(Rothstein 2009: 86)

He goes on to put the burden of evidence on Goldberg, his disputant, to offer evidence that public health solutions to such social problems would indeed be effective (Rothstein 2009: 86). At this point the evidence now exists for those who seek it. Recruiting pediatricians as public health allies in disseminating messages about the importance of firearm safety increases safe firearm storage (Barkin et al. 2008). India has been pursuing an ambitious urban re-development program, aiming to make the country "slum-free," in order to simultaneously improve "housing, water supply, sanitation[,] ... education, health and social security" (Ministry of Urban Housing and Poverty Alleviation 2010: 1). As elaborated in the case study at the end of this chapter, I have previously argued that the empirical data on climate change communication indicates that climate change messages become more compelling when reframed as "public health" matters (Valles 2015). But this is only a cursory sampling of a few examples; resources such as the 2008 WHO social determinants report provide a plethora of evidence for how many social reforms can be, have been, and should be pursued as public health matters (of course, not to the exclusion of other reasons for favoring housing reform, etc.) (Commission on Social Determinants of Health 2008).

Health in All Policies, as a model and an ethos, has been widely adopted for decades, though it appears newer since the label did not catch on until the mid-2000s. The Lalonde Report had urged coordinated health promotion policies, ranging from healthcare policies to rewriting laws regulating impaired driving to boosting public physical recreation facilities (Lalonde 1974). The Declaration of Alma-Ata pointed to intersectoral collaboration for improving health (International Conference on Primary Health Care 1978). By 1986, the year of the Ottawa Charter, WHO's governing body had adopted "intersectoral actions for health" as its favored methodology (World Health Organization 1986a). Two years later, that notion was formulated as a program of action—dubbed "Healthy Public Policy"—advocating for "an explicit concern for health and equity in all areas of policy" (Second International Conference on Health Promotion 1988). In the 2000s, "Health in All Policies" gave a new name to the old model (Ståhl et al. 2006). The model itself remains substantially the same, and the "Health in All Policies" literature is quite open about this (Centers for Disease Control and Prevention 2015).

It is now the norm for a wide array of agents—with or without government mandate—to promote population health, and to do so through a wide range of policies and initiatives. The Sioux Water Protectors featured in Chapter 2 took up the fight for their population health and control over their social determinants of health in a fight *against* government intervention. In the private sector, workplaces have been instituting effective stress-management programs as a means of promoting employee populations' wellness, reducing absenteeism, improving blood pressure, and other benefits (Richardson and Rothstein 2008). Population health science, as a research endeavor, is, to a large extent, led by the non-profit Robert Wood Johnson Foundation, filling the need left by governments and WHO (see Chapter 6) (Gottlieb et al. 2016).

Broad models of public/population health intervention, including far more than state-sponsored exercises of power, are nothing new. It is way past the time for making predictions of potential harms from a wide population health mandate via efforts in the mode of "Health in All Policies." Critics will instead need to actually point out some real harms from such policies—the historical record now exists. I do not deny that there are dire trends in health today, including disease mongering and the medicalization of normal human variation (see, for example, my critique of the inappropriate medicalization of short stature in Valles 2012). It is especially important to recognize that such hegemonic attempts to medicalize human differences (e.g., being short) have typically been the products of biomedical concepts of health being used to propose new pathologies, typically accompanied by profitable new biomedical treatments for the pathologies (González-Moreno et al. 2015).

Narrowly restricting health interventions to the prevention/treatment of diseases has not stopped hegemonic tendencies in the biomedical model—there are always new pieces of human life to be pathologized, new diseases to propose (invent?), and costly new pills to make it all better. Even the narrowest biomedical model of what health is and what can be claimed as the domain of health professionals cannot prevent creative and perhaps profit-driven hegemony. This makes it at least a little counterintuitive to worry that a population health-style broad model of health promotion is the more dangerously hegemonic option. Population health thinking is more responsible for fighting such trends than causing them, as pointed out in Arah's aforementioned rebuttal to philosophers who assume that an expansive concept of health must imply an expansion of healthcare (Arah 2009). As shown in Chapter 2, population health science is firmly rooted in the lessons of the Lalonde Report (1974), McKeown (1976), the Black Report (Black et al. 1980), and other sobering lessons that inflating the healthcare sector is woefully inadequate as a means of effectively promoting health—even aside from the other negative repercussions.

The epistemic risks of erring on the side of wide vs. narrow boundaries for public health

Should we pursue a broad model of public/population health or a narrow one? A choice either way is necessarily ethically loaded since the answer sets the scope of appropriate professional conduct. Is it inappropriate for public health organizations to officially advocate for fair wage laws as necessary health measures? Would it be professionally inappropriate for them to *not* do so? I have made the case for why a broad model is desirable and appropriate. But for those readers who might still be unconvinced, I urge them to consider the epistemic risks at stake—the risks of either erring on the side of too broad a model or too narrow a model. In the face of dispute over how much we need to worry about constraining and enforcing the boundaries of population health science's scope of research and action, we would be better off adopting the temporary strategy of going broad even while the dispute continues.

Heather Douglas inspired an active philosophical literature on science and values by reviving the oft-forgotten lesson that when we make inferences based on uncertain evidence, we must proceed in light of not only the weight of the evidence, but also considerations of what would happen if we made the wrong inference: the "inductive risk" (Douglas 2000). Biddle more recently extended this to the more general "epistemic risk ... the risk of being wrong" (Biddle 2016: 202) and Biddle and Kukla have surveyed the geography of the expansive terrain of epistemic risk (Biddle and Kukla 2017). The question, here, is whether to steer toward a broad program or narrow program of public/population health in light of the available evidence, and in light of considering the potential repercussions for choosing one model or the other. In other words, would it be safer to err on the side of narrowness or broadness in the public health promotion domain? The safer bet, it seems to me, is to err on the side of a broader scope.

The foremost reason why I am so sanguine about the broad public health model, as described above, is that the model has not caused the feared calamities despite being in operation for decades. Where are these calamities? Could there be future unknown risks of choosing too broad a model? There is a deep-seated conservatism beneath the suggestions that we should favor a narrow model of public health as government intervention balanced with the interests of individual citizens—the model that dominated the twentieth-century public health theory and that inspired pushback from population health science and from social medicine (among others) (Evans et al. 1994; Anderson et al. 2005). That conservatism is perhaps best displayed in Epstein's full-throated defense of the narrow model as an expression of classical liberalism (Epstein 2003). He includes a rejection of Marmot's calls for economic reforms to decrease the steep slope of the health–wealth gradient, saying that inequalities are surely a necessary consequence of the gradual health and economic gains across the globe (Epstein 2003). Historian Richard Novak's reply declines to choose between broad vs. narrow public health, but systematically takes apart Epstein's and others' ahistorical and positive—even romantic—views of what classical public health was and did (Novak 2003). The narrow old model of public health not only comfortably coexisted with the horrific inequities (health and otherwise) of US Jim Crow segregation laws, but even served as a potent tool of oppression against women, minorities, and other marginalized populations deemed public health threats and hence subjected to involuntary sterilization, abusive policing, discriminatory quarantines, callous destruction of housing deemed unsanitary, etc. (Novak 2003). This serves as a sobering historical reminder that a narrow model of public health as government authorized action is not necessarily less potent in its individual actions—it just intensely focuses health promotion efforts on certain targets.

Returning to the question I posed above about fair wage laws, the public health community has decidedly come down on the side of lending its collective professional voice to calls for a living wage, under the quite intuitive rationale that public health requires members of the public to … live. Similarly, I am heartened to see medical organizations speaking out against gun-ridden communities (American Pediatric Association et al. 2016). Broadbent and Epstein single out Michael Marmot for pressing too ambitiously broad a population health promotion agenda, but Marmot's WHO commission spends much of its report devoted to precisely illustrating the available data on horrible health inequities, explaining that these indefensible patterns must be changed, and recommending how. For instance, rural populations are afflicted by health-harming social injustices, and we must remediate the injustices: "counter the inequitable consequences of urban growth through action that addresses rural land tenure and rights and ensures rural livelihoods that support healthy living, adequate investment in rural infrastructure, and policies that support rural-to-urban migrants" (Commission on Social Determinants of Health 2008: 4).

I acknowledge the risk of health considerations overtaking other considerations when policymakers weigh the costs and benefits of proposals such as the aforementioned living wage laws, though it is important to keep in mind that the efforts of Health in All Policies are meant as a corrective to the unacceptable *absence* of health considerations during non-healthcare policymaking (Rudolph et al. 2013). The proposal is not to elevate health considerations above all other considerations. One key suggestion is that we should routinely take measures such as drafting "health impact assessments" for all manner of policies (Rudolph et al. 2013), allowing us to anticipate the health consequences of policies, based on the hard-learned lesson sketched in Chapter 2: the causes of health and disease are distributed throughout every corner social life. It would be foolish to make policies such as farming regulations without expecting consequences for the relevant population's diet and health. Myopic policymakers could choose their priorities poorly and consider health implications over and above considerations such as economic stability, but the reverse seems far more likely given past experience. The particular risk of having health outcomes overtake policymaking considerations is a problem partly shared across all policy contexts in the age of "evidence-based policy" and its attendant risks of setting improper success metrics, as illustrated in a 2012 book by philosopher Nancy Cartwright and economist Jeremy Hardie (Cartwright and Hardie 2012). There is by no means an overabundance of attention to the health impacts of urban planning, agricultural regulation, early childhood education, firearms regulation, etc. The same goes for climate change, as examined in this chapter's upcoming case study.

The dangers arising from broad public health promotion efforts are serious, though they are dangers that arise in any public health intervention, broad or narrow: stigmatization, coercion, cultural imperialism, etc. For instance, public health nutrition's conceptualization of obesity has been panned as irresponsibly stigmatizing or victim-blaming (Adler and Stewart 2009). In a similar vein, Buetow and Docherty strive to keep population health considerations from intruding into primary care, in part because of cases such as previous misguided public health messages about weight loss and health (Buetow and Docherty 2005), though evidentiary errors occur across all health evidence including the constantly evolving practices of primary care. We can always misjudge interventions based on the available evidence. And, whether it is gun control laws or childhood vaccinations, inappropriate methods of implementing health promotion interventions can be exceedingly harmful even when the underlying evidence is solid. Coggon is right that paternalism is "at the heart" of public health ethics concerns over the proper role of the state (Coggon 2012: xiv)—we must prevent the state from playing the metaphorical role of a condescending father figure. Yet, non-state actors, such as physicians, are just as capable of being paternalistic (Childress 1982)—paternalism is the expression of an improper power balance, and as a result any powerful agent among the distributed agents of population health can act improperly and paternalistically. The risks of abusive expressions of power are ever-present in all unequal power relationships across social life— that is a fact of social life that is no different whether one adopts a narrow public health model or a broad public/population health model. But, given the choice between the narrow model of public health vs. the broader one, the latter option is better suited to preventing unacceptable social repercussions. The broad model of population health, after all, is the model that is committed to looking for and addressing social dynamics that harm well-being. Most importantly, it is committed to doing so in participatory and collaborative ways (McQueen et al. 2012a; World Health Organization 2015; Rudolph et al. 2013). If we are going to err on the side of veering too narrow or too broad in public health, let it be too broad.

Conclusion: expanding philosophy of population health to catch up with science and practice

In this chapter, I have argued that the philosophers of public health have erred by policing the boundary between things that are vs. aren't public health matters. Instead, I make the positive philosophical case for doing population health promotion free of such preset boundaries. To use the terminology currently favored in the population health community, I make the philosophical case for pursuing "Health in All Policies." I have reviewed objections to such broad models of public health—primarily coming from the philosophical community. The concerns suggest a need to keep health promotion activities constrained in order to keep health concepts and the healthcare sector from growing amorphous or hegemonic, to the detriment of health and well-being. Building on earlier philosophical work (Arah 2009; Goldberg 2014), I rebut the claims that knocking down the boundaries of public health—as population health science does— commits neither a philosophical overreach nor a practical overreach.

It is worth pointing out here population health theorist Kindig's reply to the concern that population health is "so broad as to include everything"—he says, "the inherent value of a population health perspective is that it facilitates integration of knowledge across the many factors that influence health and health outcomes" (Kindig 2010). A broad model of public health such as the one embraced by population health science can seem absurd for trying to deal with everything—but advocates of such models only pursue them because the empirical evidence has led them to recognize that the causes of health are distributed across all social life (see Chapter 2).

Population health science is expansive in its scope, but one can accept this scope without endorsing arrogance or hegemony by health experts—quite the opposite. Chapter 2 showed the intellectual crisis created by the gradual recognition that the branches of health outcomes in society are more twisted and tangled than initially recognized, and that the roots of its social causes are similarly tangled, reaching far deeper than anticipated. Population health urges that we think holistically about the complete and baffling whole of the gnarled tree of a population's health. Such a call for big-picture thinking is both an expression of bold optimism ("we can do better!") and humbling admission that no single entity can understand or tend to the tree alone. Each person, each sector of society (including government), each measure, and each health discipline offers "only a part and not the whole" (Kindig 2010).

I have argued that attempts to limit the scope of what should be done in the name of health promotion are unwise, not least because they are belied by the historical record. Operationalizing a broad population health model by promoting some version of a "Health in All Policies" perspective dates back to at least the 1970s (Lalonde 1974). So far the effects have been overwhelmingly positive, making it all the stranger to see predictions of potential harm from the hypothetical adoption of such models. Philosophy of public health will need to contend with the fact that a broad model of public health has become the dominant view among scholars of public health and population health. Chapter 5 (the second half of Section 2) will continue this argument by showing that innovations in how causation is conceptualized in population health science give us additional reasons to favor a broad model of health promotion.

Chapter 5 will examine causation in population health, and the challenge of picking the right causes and the right effects to examine and to intervene upon, out of the massive network of causes and effects in health. The chapter will prominently feature the "Fundamental Cause Theory" of health, developed by Bruce Link and Jo Phelan, which arose out of the same historical milieu as the wider population health framework (1990s attempts to think broadly about health and its "upstream" causes in social life); Goldberg cites this same model in his philosophical dismantling of the boundary problem (Link and Phelan 1995; Goldberg 2014). Link and Phelan argue, one key contribution that health experts should bring to policy debates is to articulate how, "minimum wage, housing for homeless people, capital-gains taxes, parenting leave, head-start programs, or other initiatives of this type" are in fact powerful health policies (for good or for ill), even though they are not widely understood to be so (Link and Phelan 1995: 90). A broad model of health promotion is tied to models showing that, *and showing how*, health outcomes are the results of broad ranges of causes.

Case study: global climate change

Global climate change is perhaps the best example of a health problem that urgently requires a broad conception of what population health is and of the range of interventions needed to promote it. The *Lancet* and University College London Institute for Global Health Commission begins its sweeping report on the topic with the declaration: "Climate change is the biggest global health threat of the 21st century" (Costello et al. 2009: 1693). Some climate change phenomena will be good for some populations (warmer average winter temperatures are appealing to me and many other residents in my northern city), but the health effects of climate change are overwhelmingly negative—populations across the globe have committed themselves to cultures within particular climatic contexts: housing materials, agricultural systems, transportation infrastructures, habits of life, etc. are all developed to work within a given climate, so a relatively rapid shift in climate threatens all such social structures. Increased rates of heat exhaustion, rising rates of waterborne diseases such as cholera, epidemics of undernutrition due to faltering agriculture, escalating mental health harms from stresses such as displaced populations, and many more harms are happening now and promise to worsen with time (Smith et al. 2014: 741). Figure 4.1 provides a simplified conceptual diagram of the relationships between climate change's causal dynamics with population health.

It is important to note here that a population health science framework is particularly well suited to addressing climate change, in part because of its ability to contend with health's temporal trends, as discussed at great length in Chapter 3. This is key because climate change ethicists have firmly established that the unique ethical challenges of climate change are in large part due to the fact that its harms are intergenerational—future generations will suffer more from our climate change behaviors than ours will (Gardiner 2001). Keyes and Galea's very definition of population health science includes the science's attention to "pathways within social interactions that develop across the life course and across generations" (Keyes and Galea 2016b: 634).

Yet, even as population health scholars from many specialties have begun focusing their attention on climate change, the topic has largely remained in the peripheral vision of bioethics and of public health ethics (exceptions include Dwyer 2009; Resnik 2012; MacPherson 2013; Valles 2015). Despite the disproportionately meager attention by philosophers, population health scholars have taken up the cause. The WHO Commission on Social Determinants of Health features climate change prominently. This is as it should be. Global climate change is a health harm that exacerbates existing health inequities.

> Climate change stands out as a priority area for attention in relation to health inequities. Climate change, urbanization, rural development, agriculture, and food security are intertwined determinants of population health and health equity.
>
> (Commission on Social Determinants of Health 2008: 196)

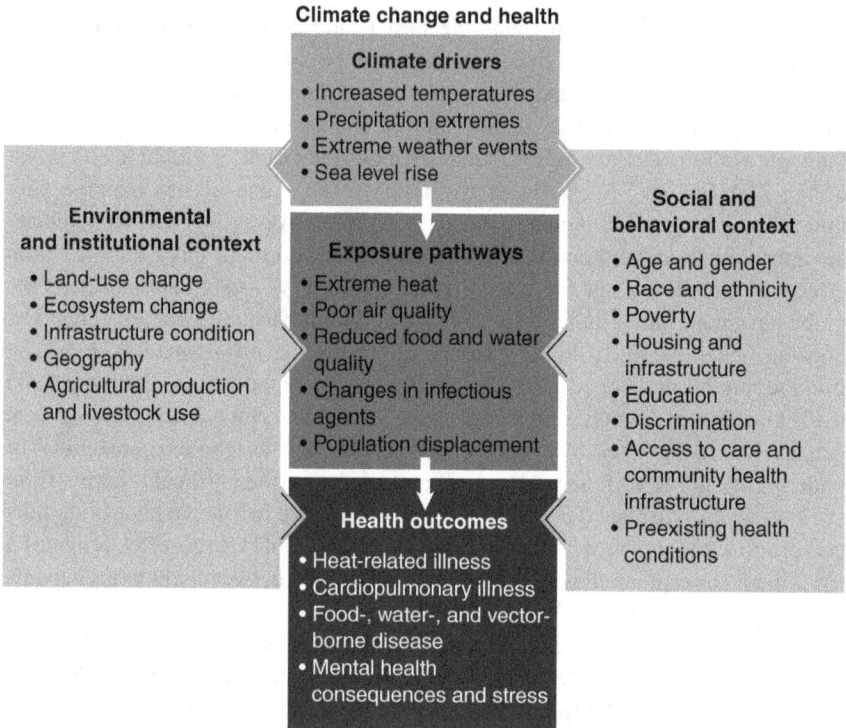

Figure 4.1 Conceptual diagram illustrating the exposure pathways by which climate change affects human health.

Source: Balbus et al. 2016: 30.

The Commission's willingness to be openly prescriptive—to explicitly take an ethical stance—is a welcome contrast to the famously non-prescriptive stance taken by the UN entity tasked with studying climate change, the Intergovernmental Panel on Climate Change (IPCC): "the work of the organization is … policy-relevant and yet policy-neutral, never policy-prescriptive" (Intergovernmental Panel on Climate Change 2016). This offers a stark parallel to the debate over the public health boundary problem. The IPCC takes the official stance of policy neutrality in much the same way that the public health discipline adopted a concept of scientific objectivity that "precluded public health from playing a more prominent role in social reform" (National Association of County & City Health Officials 2014: 8). Population health science scholars, along with many likeminded others in areas related to public health, have largely abandoned that restrictive view of the boundaries of which debates they may engage with or whether they may offer recommendations in addition to assessments.

The relative neglect of climate change by philosophers of health is partly a consequence of entrenched conceptions of the boundaries around public health.

Rothstein and Powers and Faden each offer lists of supposed public health problems that seem dubious to them for boundary problem reasons: Rothstein cites "environmental degradation" (Rothstein 2009: 86) and Powers and Faden cite "environmental and occupational hazards" (Powers and Faden 2006: 10). It should then come as no surprise that there is a scarcity of public health ethics literature on climate change if there is theoretically grounded doubt that climate change is even a public health problem. This relative neglect has largely left climate change dialogue to continue being framed "as an environmental problem" but not a "public health problem" (Myers et al. 2012: 1106).

By overemphasizing climate change as an environmental problem (a threat to abstract ecosystems, non-human species, etc.—that is, climate-change-as-threat-to-polar-bears), non-experts have been given too little motivation to take climate change seriously (Valles 2015). A reason for optimism, as I point out in a 2015 article (Valles 2015), is that framing climate change as a public health problem seems to reduce public skepticism and apathy about the problem. Maibach et al. see their empirical data on climate messages as suggesting that the existing credibility of public health experts would lend credibility and urgency to climate change messages, rather than risking the existing credibility of those public health experts. Presenting climate change as a public health problem:

> should help people make connections to already familiar problems such as asthma, allergies, and infectious diseases experienced in their communities … The frame also presents the opportunity to involve additional trusted communication partners on the issue, notably public health experts and local community leaders.
>
> (Maibach et al. 2010: 299)

Follow-up research similarly suggests that public health experts are well positioned to be trusted sources of information about climate change. Curiously, it turns out that (in the disproportionately well-studied US population, at least), people trust their primary care physicians above all other sources of information about climate change's health impacts (Maibach et al. 2015).

The upcoming chapter on health causation will center much of its attention on Link and Phelan's "Fundamental Cause Theory," a model for understanding the social factors (e.g., money) that serve as the underlying causes of a multitude of different positive and negative population health patterns. A recent article (co-authored by Link) considers the bioethical dimensions of how and why physicians desperately need to be better educated in "structural competency"—their understanding of how patients' health is shaped by factors outside the healthcare domain, such as exposure to a pollution in one's workplace (Reich et al. 2016). They argue that physicians must understand and even attempt to intervene in the underlying causes of their patients' health. In light of Maibach et al.'s findings about patients' trust in their physicians as sources of climate change health information and Reich et al.'s ethical exhortations, it seems that there is a pressing need for physicians to participate in the population health science endeavor to address climate change's health impacts.

The prospect of involving physicians more thoroughly in public/population health social policy deliberations reinvites the hegemony concern—it is important to consider whether physicians and other healthcare experts might end up monopolizing the deliberations. Moreover, to reiterate Arah's point cited above, it is philosophically and practically vital that we avoid conflating health problems with healthcare problems (Arah 2009). The key in this case is that Reich et al. recommend involving physicians in social policy matters (e.g., climate change) not as commanders, but as participants in a massive multiparty process in which they have a professional stake, by virtue of their obligations to care for patients. Physicians are important participants in the collaborative efforts of Health in All Policies (Rudolph et al. 2013).

Even if physicians and other health experts were to vastly expand their interest in climate change, the multidimensionality of climate change is so abundantly clear to all experts in the area that it seems entirely implausible that health or healthcare would become conceptually or practically hegemonic in climate change discourse. I have made a case for why the boundary problem isn't much of a problem at all, though I am sympathetic with the concerns of those who worry about the boundary problem. So much is at stake that we must proceed carefully. Given my above points about epistemic risk, proceeding carefully means that we should favor a broad model of public/population health. The global climate change case study serves as an illustration of what happens when the population health aspects of a problem are not well understood by policy-makers, the public, or even the philosophers who can help serve as intermediaries between those groups and population health science practitioners.

Works cited

Adler, N. E. and Stewart, J. (2009) Reducing obesity: Motivating action while not blaming the victim. *Milbank Quarterly* 87, 49–70.

American Pediatric Association, American Academy of Pediatrics, American Academy of Pediatrics, et al. (2016) *Dear Senator*. Available at: www.apha.org/~/media/files/pdf/advocacy/letters/2016/160617_ph_senate_gvp_amdts.ashx.

Anderson, M. R., Smith, L. and Sidel, V. W. (2005) What is social medicine? *Monthly Review*, 56.

Arah, O. A. (2009) On the relationship between individual and population health. *Medicine, Health Care and Philosophy* 12, 235–244.

Balbus, J., Crimmins, A., Gamble, J. L., et al. (2016) Introduction: Climate Change and Human Health. In: U.S. Global Change Research Program (ed.) *The Impacts of Climate Change on Human Health in the United States: A Scientific Assessment.* Washington D. C.

Barkin, S. L., Finch, S. A., Ip, E. H., et al. (2008) Is office-based counseling about media use, timeouts, and firearm storage effective? Results from a cluster-randomized, controlled trial. *Pediatrics* 122, e15–e25.

Bell, K. (2017) *Health and Other Unassailable Values: Reconfigurations of Health, Evidence and Ethics.* London: Routledge.

Biddle, J. B. (2016) Inductive risk, epistemic risk, and overdiagnosis of disease. *Perspectives on Science* 24, 192–205.

Biddle, J. B. and Kukla, R. (2017) The Geography of Epistemic Risk. In: Elliott, K. C. and Richards, T. (eds) *Exploring Inductive Risk: Case Studies of Values in Science.* New York: Oxford University Press, 215–238.

Black, D., Morris, J., Smith, C. and Townsend, P. (1980) Inequalities in Health: Report of a Research Working Group on Inequalities in Health. London: Department of Health and Social Security.

Broadbent, A. (2013) *Philosophy of Epidemiology.* New York: Palgrave Macmillan.

Buetow, S. and Docherty, B. (2005) The seduction of general practice and illegitimate birth of an expanded role in population health care. *Journal of Evaluation in Clinical Practice* 11, 397–404.

Callahan, D. (1973) The WHO definition of "health." *The Hastings Center Report* 1, 77–87.

Cartwright, N. and Hardie, J. (2012) *Evidence-Based Policy: A Practical Guide to Doing It Better.* New York: Oxford University Press.

Centers for Disease Control and Prevention. (2015) *Health in All Policies.* Available at: www.cdc.gov/policy/hiap/resources/.

Childress, J. F. (1982) *Who Should Decide?: Paternalism in Health Care.* New York: Oxford University Press.

Coggon, J. (2012) *What Makes Health Public? A Critical Evaluation of Moral, Legal, and Political Claims in Public Health.* New York: Cambridge University Press.

Commission on Social Determinants of Health. (2008) Closing the Gap in a Generation: Health Equity Through Action on the Social Determinants of Health. Geneva: World Health Organization.

Costello, A., Abbas, M., Allen, A., et al. (2009) Managing the health effects of climate change. *Lancet* 373, 1693–1733.

Douglas, H. (2000) Inductive risk and values in science. *Philosophy of Science* 67, 559–579.

Dwyer, J. (2009) How to connect bioethics and environmental ethics: Health, sustainability, and justice. *Bioethics* 23, 497–502.

Epstein, R. A. (2003) Let the shoemaker stick to his last: A defense of the "old" public health. *Perspectives in Biology and Medicine* 46, S138–S159.

Evans, R. G., Barer, M. L. and Marmor, T. R. (1994) *Why Are Some People Healthy and Others Not? The Determinants of Health of Populations.* New York: Aldine De Gruyter.

Gardiner, S. M. (2001) The real tragedy of the commons. *Philosophy & Public Affairs* 30, 387–416.

Goldberg, D. S. (2009) In support of a broad model of public health: Disparities, social epidemiology and public health causation. *Public Health Ethics* 2, 70–83.

Goldberg, D. S. (2014) The implications of fundamental cause theory for priority setting. *American Journal of Public Health* 104, 1839–1843.

González-Moreno, M., Saborido, C. and Teira, D. (2015) Disease-mongering through clinical trials. *Studies in History and Philosophy of Biological and Biomedical Sciences* 51, 11–18.

Gottlieb, L., Glymour, M. M., Kersten, E., et al. (2016) Challenges to an integrated population health research agenda: Targets, scale, tradeoffs and timing. *Social Science & Medicine* 150, 279–285.

Hagedorn, J., Paras, C. A., Greenwich, H. and Hagopian, A. (2016) The role of labor unions in creating working conditions that promote public health. *American Journal of Public Health* 106, 989–995.

Harris, D., Puskarz, K. and Golab, C. (2016) Population health: Curriculum framework for an emerging discipline. *Population health management* 19, 39–45.

Hausman, D. M. (2015) *Valuing Health: Well-Being, Freedom and Suffering.* New York: Oxford University Press.

Health Research & Educational Trust. (2015) Approaches to Population Health in 2015: A National Survey of Hospitals. Chicago: Health Research & Educational Trust.

Holland, S. (2015) *Public Health Ethics.* Malden, MA: Polity Press.

Intergovernmental Panel on Climate Change. (2016) *Organization.* Available at: www.ipcc.ch/organization/organization.shtml.

International Conference on Primary Health Care. (1978) Declaration of Alma-Ata. Alma-Ata, Kazakhstan.

Katikireddi, S. V. and Valles, S. A. (2015) Coupled ethical-epistemic analysis of public health research and practice: Categorizing variables to improve population health and equity. *American Journal of Public Health* 105, e36–e42.

Keyes, K. M. and Galea, S. (2016a) *Population Health Science.* New York: Oxford University Press.

Keyes, K. M. and Galea, S. (2016b) Setting the agenda for a new discipline: Population health science. *American Journal of Public Health* 106, 633–634.

Kindig, D. (2010) *What Is Population Health?* Available at: www.improvingpopulation-health.org/blog/what-is-population-health.html.

King, M., Smith, A. and Gracey, M. (2009) Indigenous Health Part 2: The underlying causes of the health gap. *The Lancet* 374, 76–85.

Kirk, D. S. and Hardy, M. (2014) The acute and enduring consequences of exposure to violence on youth mental health and aggression. *Justice Quarterly* 31, 539–567.

Lalonde, M. (1974) *A New Perspective on the Health of Canadians.* Ottawa, Canada: Health and Welfare Canada.

Link, B. G. and Phelan, J. (1995) Social conditions as fundamental causes of disease. *Journal of Health and Social Behavior* 35, 80–94.

MacPherson, C. C. (2013) Climate change is a bioethics problem. *Bioethics* 27, 305–308.

Maibach, E. W., Kreslake, J. M., Roser-Renouf, C., et al. (2015) Do Americans understand that global warming is harmful to human health? Evidence from a national survey. *Annals of Global Health* 81, 396–409.

Maibach, E. W., Nisbet, M., Baldwin, P., et al. (2010) Reframing climate change as a public health issue: An exploratory study of public reactions. *BMC Public Health* 10, 299.

Marmot, M. (2006) Health in an unequal world: Social circumstances, biology and disease. *Clinical Medicine* 6, 559–572.

McKeown, T. (1976) *The Role of Medicine: Dream, Mirage, or Nemesis.* London: Nuffield Provincial Hospitals Trust.

McQueen, D. V., Wismar, M., Lin, V. and Jones, C. M. (2012a) Introduction: Health in All Policies, the Social Determinants of Health and Governance. In: McQueen, D. V., Wismar, M., Lin, V., et al. (eds) *Intersectoral Governance for Health in All Policies: Structures, Actions and Experiences.* Copenhagen: WHO Regional Office for Europe.

McQueen, D. V., Wismar, M., Lin, V., et al. (2012b) *Intersectoral Governance for Health in All Policies: Structures, Actions and Experiences.* Copenhagen: WHO Regional Office for Europe.

Metzl, J. and Kirkland, A. (2010) *Against Health: How Health Became the New Morality*. New York: New York University Press.

Meyer, I. H. and Schwartz, S. (2000) Social issues as public health: Promise and peril. *American Journal of Public Health* 90, 1189–1191.

Ministry of Urban Housing and Poverty Alleviation. (2010) *Rajiv Awas Yojana: Guidelines for slum-free city planning*. New Delhi: Ministry of Urban Housing and Poverty Alleviation,.

Myers, T. A., Nisbet, M. C., Maibach, E. W. and Leiserowitz, A. A. (2012) A public health frame arouses hopeful emotions about climate change. *Climatic Change* 113, 1105–1112.

Nash, D. B., Fabius, R. J., Skoufalos, A., et al. (2016) *Population Health: Creating a Culture of Wellness*. Second ed. Burlington, MA: Jones & Bartlett Learning.

National Association of County & City Health Officials. (2014) Expanding the Boundaries: Health Equity and Public Health Practice. Washington, DC: National Association of County & City Health Officials.

Novak, W. J. (2003) Private wealth and public health: A critique of Richard Epstein's defense of the "old" public health. *Perspectives in Biology and Medicine* 46, S176-S198.

Ohri-Vachaspati, P., Isgor, Z., Rimkus, L., et al. (2015) Child-directed marketing inside and on the exterior of fast-food restaurants. *American Journal of Preventive Medicine* 48, 22–30.

Powers, M. and Faden, R. R. (2006) *Social Justice: The Moral Foundations of Public Health and Health Policy*. New York: Oxford University Press.

Reich, A. D., Hansen, H. B. and Link, B. G. (2016) Fundamental interventions: How clinicians can address the fundamental causes of disease. *Journal of Bioethical Inquiry* 13, 185–192.

Resnik, D. B. (2012) *Environmental Health Ethics*. Cambridge: Cambridge University Press.

Richardson, K. M. and Rothstein, H. R. (2008) Effects of occupational stress management intervention programs: A meta-analysis. *Journal of Occupational Health Psychology* 13, 69–93.

Rothstein, M. A. (2002) Rethinking the meaning of public health. *The Journal of Law, Medicine & Ethics* 30, 144–149.

Rothstein, M. A. (2009) The limits of public health: A response. *Public Health Ethics* 2, 84–88.

Rudolph, L., Caplan, J., Ben-Moshe, K. and Dillon, L. (2013) Health in All Policies: A Guide for State and Local Governments. Washington, DC: American Public Health Association and Public Health Institute.

Scheper-Hughes, N. (2014) The house gun: White writing, white fears and black justice. *Anthropology Today* 30, 8–12.

Schramme, T. (2016) The metric and the threshold problem for theories of health justice: A comment on Venkatapuram. *Bioethics* 30, 19–24.

Second International Conference on Health Promotion. (1988) Healthy Public Policy: Report on the Adelaide Conference. Adelaide, Australia: World Health Organization.

Sholl, J. (2017) The muddle of medicalization: Pathologizing or medicalizing? *Theoretical Medicine and Bioethics* 38, 265–278.

Sidorov, J. and Romney, M. (2016) The Spectrum of Care. In: Nash, D. B., Fabius, R. J., Skoufalos, A., et al. (eds) *Population Health: Creating a Culture of Wellness*. Second ed. Burlington, MA: Jones & Bartlett Learning, 19–41.

Smith, K. R., Woodward, A., Campbell-Lendrum, D., et al. (2014) Human Health: Impacts, Adaptation, and Co-benefits. In: Field, C. B., Barros, V. R., Dokken, D. J., et al. (eds) *Climate Change 2014: Impacts, Adaptation, and Vulnerability. Part A: Global and Sectoral Aspects. Contribution of Working Group II to the Fifth Assessment Report of the Intergovernmental Panel on Climate Change.* Cambridge: Cambridge University Press, 709–754.

Ståhl, T., Wismar, M., Ollila, E., et al. (2006) *Health in All Policies: Prospects and Potentials.* Finland: Finnish Ministry of Social Affairs and Health.

The Public Policy Advisory Network on Female Genital Surgeries in Africa. (2012) Seven things to know about female genital surgeries in Africa. *Hastings Center Report* 42, 19–27.

Valles, S. A. (2012) Lionel Penrose and the concept of normal variation in human intelligence. *Studies in History and Philosophy of Biological and Biomedical Sciences* 43, 231–289.

Valles, S. A. (2015) Bioethics and the framing of climate change's health risks. *Bioethics* 29, 334–341.

Valles, S. A. (2016) *Politics and the Other Lead Poisoning: The Public Health Ethics of Gun Violence.* Available at: https://msubioethics.com/2016/11/17/public-health-ethics-of-gun-violence/.

Venkatapuram, S. (2011) *Health Justice: An Argument from the Capabilities Approach.* Malden, MA: Polity Press.

World Health Organization. (1986a) Intersectoral action for health: The role of intersectoral cooperation in national strategies for health for all. Geneva: World Health Organization.

World Health Organization. (1986b) Ottawa Charter for Health Promotion. Ottawa, ON: World Health Organization.

World Health Organization. (2015) Health in All Policies Training Manual. Geneva: World Health Organization.

Young, T. K. (2005) *Population Health: Concepts and Methods.* New York: Oxford University Press.

5 Prioritizing the right population health causes and effects

Introduction: addressing population health problems at the roots

> A focus only on indicators of health "within the skin" has the disadvantage that upstream interventions tend to be ignored as lying outside the health domain, consigning population health research to remaining at the level of describing *what* but not analyzing *why*.
>
> (McDowell et al. 2004: 391)

The philosophical issues in health causation are closely related to the philosophical issues in the appropriate reach of health promotion activities (Chapter 4), which are in turn closely related to questions of health's meaning (Chapter 3), which is embedded in the contingencies of a population's social life (Chapter 2). Health is a life course trajectory of complete well-being in social context, and health promotion activities must correspondingly extend into every corner of social life. One danger here is that if population health science is virtually unlimited in its scope of concern, its attention could become problematically diluted. The dynamics of individual health, population health and social life are causally bound up together ... Now what? Trying to understand and/or intervene upon every causal relationship would be impossible and foolish. Which causes ought we to prioritize? I write this chapter on philosophy of health causation after taking to heart Dowdy and Pai's warning that "academic epidemiology is evolving into a scientific discipline with increasing focus on objectivity and on education in methods to deduce causality," when what the world most needs are "scientists with integrative knowledge-translating skill sets": "accountable health advocates" (Dowdy and Pai 2012: 914). As Galea puts it, "an activist role ... is unavoidable if one aspires to promote population health" (Galea 2018: 227). Which philosophy of causation best serves the practical project of facilitating effective health action in the real world? This chapter offers some recommendations.

This chapter is not about philosophy of population health causation in general, but rather the more particular challenge of prioritizing the right population health causes and effects. It brings a philosophical perspective to population health science's efforts to sort through the overabundance of health causes and effects in the world. The chapter largely contrasts my philosophy of population health causation with Alex Broadbent's pioneering book, *Philosophy of Epidemiology* (Broadbent 2013). First, I endorse Fundamental Cause Theory as a particularly promising contribution to population health science (Link and Phelan 1995). "Fundamental causes" (e.g., "money" or "prestige") are flexible social resources that manifest a unique type of stability—their presence or absence will engender effects that are predictably positive or negative, but will cause their positive or negative effects via wildly different health mechanisms and outcomes. I then proceed to review the objections Broadbent raises to the unreflective use of "risk factors" in the public health literature, and contrast those objections to the different objections raised in the population health science literature. I show how the latter objections lead us away from Broadbent's solution of refining our models of how individual cases of disease are caused and instead focus on the causes of the variations in disease incidence between populations. The chapter then argues for the value of shifting at least some attention away from tracing the causation of individual diseases and instead directing it toward tracing the causation of health—"salutogenesis" (Mittelmark et al. 2017). The chapter's case study illustrates the suggestions from above using the case of Brazil's HIV/AIDS response.

"Fundamental Cause Theory"

Bruce Link and Jo Phelan, in a widely cited 1995 article and later follow-up work, argue that certain social determinants of health—"money, power, prestige," etc.—are not just causally relevant to epidemiology—they are "fundamental causes" (Link and Phelan 1995; Phelan and Link 2005; Phelan et al. 2010; Reich et al. 2016; Phelan and Link 2015). They elaborate that understanding proximate causes of disease can (obviously) help in improving populations' health, but "if one genuinely wants to alter the effects of a fundamental cause, one must address the fundamental cause itself" (Link and Phelan 1995: 88). They explain fundamental causes are social resources that each increase/decrease ability to avoid health harms (Link and Phelan 1995). Resources are flexible, so their presence/absence will affect many health outcomes via many mechanisms (Link and Phelan 1995). Disease risks are various and changing, but flexible resources are helpful across most such risks (Link and Phelan 1995).

Fundamental causes are philosophically challenging to grasp because they are variable in their effects and pathways thereto, even to the point of seeming paradoxical. Take the case of body weight and its attendant health effects. In high-income countries, poverty is a cause of being overweight (Nguyen et al. 2015). But in lower-income countries (including in the not-too-distant past of currently high-income countries), poverty causes underweight. Today, many low- and middle-income countries have seen their high rates of poverty generate dual epidemics: health problems related to overweight in some subpopulations and health problems related to underweight in other subpopulations of the same country, all while the mechanisms for these double-edged epidemics remain unclear (Manyanga et al. 2014). Fundamental Cause Theory helps to make sense of such bizarre phenomena, showing there is nothing paradoxical about poverty having two opposite effects. Different populations of impoverished people will suffer from different health harms because they lack the buffering effect of money, and this can even include opposite problems in the case of body weight; sometimes poverty forces one to go hungry and other times it forces one to eat foods that supply a surplus of calories but a poor balance of macro- and micro-nutrients. We don't always know how the mechanisms of the harms operate, but we can be quite confident that the prevalence of weight problems in impoverished populations are indeed traceable to poverty. And, in turn, we can be confident that directly fighting poverty would ameliorate these and many other health problems (Doku and Neupane 2015).

As discussed in Chapter 2, Marmot et al. stumbled upon a particularly illustrative example of the effect that socioeconomic status has on health in his Whitehall Study (Marmot et al. 1984), and it was only through the accumulation of similar data in other populations across the globe that it became clear the health–wealth gradient is ubiquitous—the wealthier are healthier (Marmot 2004). Fundamental Cause Theory helps to conceptualize the persistence of that effect (money offers a buffer against whichever specific health harms afflict a particular population) and also helps us to see that money is not the only such buffer, since factors such as stigma and racism can operate in analogous ways (they are also social factors that buffer some from harm while leaving others exposed).

Unfortunately, the term "fundamental cause" is misleading. There is nothing about fundamental causes that earns them the distinction of being inherently fundamental in any common understanding of the word. They are not necessarily the most upstream causes, the most basic, the lowest in their level of complexity, the most temporally prior, or otherwise unique by virtue of their fundamentality. We can debate all day if and how property rights, capitalist economics, individualism, or some other cause is somehow the fundamental cause behind poverty, but the value of investigating poverty as a fundamental cause does not depend on it being the one true genesis of resource deprivations and their effects. Instead, the importance of "fundamental causes" as targets for research and intervention stems from their unique form of *stability* as population health causes. "Fundamental causes" are flexible social buffers, and the presence or absence of these buffers is relatively consistent in the production of either net positive or net negative effects on health, though the particular benefits or harms will vary enormously in the specific health outcomes, and the mechanisms by which those health outcomes are affected will vary by time and place.

"Fundamental causes": paramount importance because of a unique type of stability

"Upstream" causes have gone by a variety of names, all attempting to get at the same problem. Birn calls for attention to the "causes of the causes of the causes"—the sources of social inequities and hence of those inequities' health effects (Birn 2009). Jones directs us to the far upstream "social determinants of equity," social factors that disproportionately distribute the social determinants of health (Jones et al. 2009). Fundamental causes have a valuable accompanying literature, but a misleading name, since the name implies that they must somehow be the final link in a causal chain. To repeat the point above, this is not what makes fundamental causes distinct and valuable, but rather the fact that fundamental causes are *flexible social buffers against health harms*. Freese and Lutfey attempt a more thorough causal analysis of the fundamental cause concept, finding more conceptual and practical importance in it than Ward's narrower analysis had found when it cashed out the theory in terms of necessary and sufficient causes (Freese and Lutfey 2011; Ward 2007). Freese and Lutfey argue that fundamental causes play a crucial explanatory task that cannot be played by other distal/distant/far upstream causes that contribute to the appearance of an effect. Fundamental causes stand out because they are not reducible to some set of more proximate/downstream causes (Freese and Lutfey 2011: 69). Racism is a fundamental cause of health, but would not qualify as such if racial dynamics could be explained away by controlling for socioeconomic status—they cannot (Freese and Lutfey 2011: 69; Phelan and Link 2015; Chetty et al. 2016).

The unique causal nature of fundamental causes becomes all the clearer when we see that James Woodward's highly regarded work on the philosophy of causation in science fails to make room for such a cause, even in a rare philosophy of science paper that gives explicit attention to epidemiology (Woodward 2010). Woodward generalizes that causal relationships that do not conform to a one-cause-one-effect pattern are relatively hazardous to manipulate due to their multitude of effects—"it will often be the case in biological or biomedical contexts that these additional effects are unwanted or deleterious" (Woodward 2010: 315). This generalization may hold in most cases, but fundamental causes deserve focused attention exactly because they do not follow this pattern. Fundamental causes are flexible social buffers against health harms. Since they operate as flexible buffers against a wide array of harms, they lack one-cause-one-effect relationships, but their effects are reliable in their *directionality*. As Link and Phelan explain: "a fundamental cause embodies a set of flexible resources, and a superior set of resources generates superior results on some outcome" (Phelan and Link 2015: 314). If we were to make headway in addressing racism, it would surely cause a plethora of "additional effects" (to use Woodward's phrase), but contra Woodward's worry about intervening in such complex causal relationships, we need not be concerned that progress against racism would yield "unwanted or deleterious" effects (Woodward 2010; Phelan and Link 2015).

We do not even have a good handle on the range of health effects that racism has now (Paradies et al. 2015), let alone the incredible diversity of effects it has in varying population contexts today or in the future. Yet, we need not sleep poorly at night for fear that the net health effects of reducing the social problem of racism will be negative. The same goes for money and other fundamental causes—the specific mechanisms and outcomes are variable and unpredictable, yet the directionality is stable: racism hurts health, poverty hurts health, etc.

While much of this chapter is devoted to contrasting my views of epidemiological causation from Broadbent's, I take it that he and I do agree that stable causal relationships are of special importance in epidemiology. The dizzying combination of variability and causal complexities makes it important for us to stay vigilant in our search for stable causal relationships that operate across these complexities. As Dammann explains, Broadbent's valuing of stability somewhat echoes both the philosophy of science concept, robustness (see, for example, Weisberg 2006), and also the concept "consistency" in Hill's famous list of factors that go into assessing whether or not a relationship is causal (Dammann 2015; Hill 1965). Applying the lessons of Link and Phelan's Fundamental Cause Theory guides us to look for special types of causal stabilities. In fundamental causes, the stability manifests in the direction of the effect—some causes are stable sources of negative health outcomes, even though the particular negative health outcomes vary enormously from context to context.

On the research level, Fundamental Cause Theory yields non-obvious and testable hypotheses, and guides research. Recent evidence indicates that education may qualify as a fundamental cause of its own, related to but distinct from prestige and money, such that "higher-educated adults" have a "personal firewall" by virtue of their relative abilities to "effectively marshal their resources (e.g., cognitive, noncognitive, social, economic) to avoid disease, disability, and premature death across vastly different contexts" (Montez et al. 2017: 1107). As a philosopher interested in epistemology—in the powers and limitations of our knowledge about health—I find Fundamental Cause Theory to be a very encouraging means of managing our vast ignorance about populations' health. Targeting fundamental causes for intervention allows us to cut through the mythical Gordian knot of our ignorance, rather than trying to untangle it. We don't know all of the harms that stigma causes in peoples' health and we don't know all of the proximate mechanisms by which those harms are generated (Hatzenbuehler et al. 2013), but we can know that tackling the upstream social problem of stigma would have health benefits that cut across the plethora of mechanisms and outcomes. Fundamental causes are causes that we can manipulate with confidence, even if we are ignorant about many aspects of the population health phenomena and their proximate causal dynamics. It is immensely important to recognize that efforts such as reducing poverty and improving education promise to solve health problems that we do not fully understand—or even problems that researchers have not yet discovered.

What is and isn't wrong with risk factors

Fundamental Cause Theory is a promising means of directing population health science toward impactful use of its limited knowledge. It is not a panacea. Crafting a philosophy of causation for population health science demands that we begin by critiquing the questions and assumptions in population health theory. Broadbent's book is exceptionally valuable in moving this process forward. One critique he offers is a careful articulation of why he is philosophically dissatisfied with the vagaries of "multifactorial thinking" dominated by "useless cataloguing of causal risk factors" (Broadbent 2013: 160). It is a critique that has been made elsewhere, but for different reasons (Krieger 1994); these reasons will be discussed below. Broadbent's account of the problems with risk factor thinking merits attention because it helps to lay out one important theoretical approach to epidemiological priorities and theoretical tools, which I will contrast with my own different set of priorities and theoretical tools.

What is wrong with risk factors? Broadbent frames the problem by fondly repeating in his book and in a subsequent article (Broadbent 2013: 148; Broadbent 2014: 253) a "lovely jibe" that Friedrich Henle ("a father of modern medicine") leveled against his theoretical opponents in 1844. Henle was a staunch advocate of the emerging germ theory's ability to offer simple and precise connections between causes and effects. Henle contrasted this with the sorts of foolish explanations that he saw other scientists offering every time they wished to explain the etiology of diseases (Broadbent 2013: 148). As Henle put it:

> poor housing and clothing, liquor and sex, hunger and anxiety. This is just as scientific as if a physicist were to teach that bodies fall because boards or beams are removed, because ropes or cables break, or because of openings, and so forth.
>
> (Henle 1844; quoted in Carter 2003, 24; Broadbent 2013: 148)

To Henle, it was not just that such social, environmental, and behavioral risk factors are explanatorily incomplete—it is that they are unscientific. Broadbent elaborates on Henle's position by explaining this is because:

> each of these kinds of causes explains only a proportion of all the cases it is cited to explain. Cataloguing risk factors for falling is unscientific, in the perfectly literal sense that it does not yield the sort of explanation that scientists who seek to explain falling seek.
>
> (Broadbent 2013: 148)

And this is the crux of Broadbent's philosophical objection—that such causes may work toward explanations of some sort, but not what he deems a proper scientific explanation:

Henle's jibe is uncomfortably applicable to modern epidemiological explanations for disease, referring as they do to a web or constellation of factors, none necessary, and many overlapping with the risk factors for other diseases.

(Broadbent 2014: 253)

Going back to Henle's analogy about the causes of falling, Broadbent argues: "the physicist is after ... a *general explanation* of falling" that explains all cases of falling, while appealing to ropes breaking can only explain some cases, boards being removed explains some other cases, etc. (Broadbent 2013: 148). So, Broadbent does not think things like poor housing are up to the task of explaining poor health in a way that he finds suitably specific, generalizable, and scientific.

Broadbent's argument pivots from there to offering a new model of what can constitute a disease, the "Contrastive Model of Disease," which rejects imprecise multifactorial "risk factor" thinking about disease causation:

SYMPTOMS Cases of D exhibit symptoms, which are absent from controls;
CASES These symptoms are caused by $C_1, \dots C_n$ together;
CONTROLS At least one of $C_1, \dots C_n$ is absent from controls.

(Broadbent 2013: 158)

Under this view, each disease must have at least one cause whose presence or absence makes the difference between having that disease or not. In other words, he redefines the criteria for what can qualify as a disease, to push scholars away from thinking of diseases only in terms of a collection of risk factors.

Henle's complaints about the state of public health science in the 1840s were reactions against the emergence of epidemiological theorists interested in social causes of disease, serving as the historical roots of contemporary research on social determinants of health, public health's professional commitment to social justice, and Health in All Policies (Ståhl et al. 2006; Krieger and Birn 1998). Indeed, the American Public Health Association includes a "Spirit of 1848 Caucus" dedicated to continuing the revolutionary social justice *zeitgeist* of the era: public health that synergizes with abolitionism, trade unionism, women's suffrage, and other related justice movements (Krieger and Birn 1998).[1] Henle tossed his 1844 barb two years after Edwin Chadwick had called attention to the effects of unsanitary living and working conditions, such as the "poor housing" ridiculed by Henle. Shortly afterward, Friedrich Engels published his own empirical study of how alcohol abuse was both a cause and an effect of disease and other miseries (Yadavendu 2014; Waitzkin 2007).[2] If we are seeking a historical figure with timeless insights into medical explanation, we would be much better off turning to Henle's contemporary and fellow pathologist, Rudolph Virchow. Even though Virchow wrongly believed bacterial infection to be an effect of diseased tissue rather than a cause, the catchphrase attributed to him, based on his views, "all diseases have two causes, one pathological, the other political," holds up very well today (Labonté et al. 2005: 6). Social determinants of health and rigorous physiological bases of disease are not in explanatory conflict with each other; they are dual complementary aspects of *every* disease.

Virchow's advice to think about both individual-level pathology and social-level health determinants partially maps onto Rose's famous distinction between the "causes of cases" and the "causes of incidence," and his advocacy for favoring the latter in population-level health promotion (Rose 1985). Rose helped to launch population health science by making this distinction between the etiology of individual cases of disease (the sorts of causal factors that Broadbent seeks) vs. the etiology of variations between populations (often social and environmental determinants). For example, many immunological and exposure factors are involved in the disease tuberculosis (TB), but infection with *Mycobacterium tuberculosis* unites all cases—this gives Broadbent exactly the sort of characteristic cause his Contrastive Model seeks. But that knowledge of the pathological etiology of cases is not all that informative for understanding what causes the *population-level* phenomenon where some groups of people have vastly higher rates of TB than others. Why do some populations have high rates of TB while other populations have low rates? The TB incidence across the globe:

> varied widely among countries in 2015, from under 10 per 100,000 population in most high-income countries to 150–300 in most of the 30 high TB burden countries ... and above 500 in a few countries including Lesotho, Mozambique and South Africa.
>
> (World Health Organization 2016a: 24)

For instance, around 4.2 percent of the US currently has latent TB—that is, is infected with *Mycobacterium tuberculosis* but is asymptomatic—yet the annual incidence of new cases of *active TB disease* is only 4.4 cases per 100,000 people (i.e. 0.0044 percent of the US population gets diagnosed with active TB disease each year) (Shea et al. 2014). What causes this massive international between-population disparity in the incidence of TB? Mainly social and environmental determinants of health, including some of the very same causes that Henle balked at: "undernutrition," housing quality, and "alcohol misuse" (World Health Organization 2016a: 104). The next section will elaborate on the significance of causes of incidence.

This brings us full circle to what is and isn't wrong with "risk factor" thinking. For Broadbent, thinking of epidemiological causation in terms of a set of risk factors, with no set of one or a few causes treated as characteristic or definitive, is wrong-headed: "... the medic ought to be after something general to say about all cases of a given disease and less interested in those causes which give rise to some cases of that disease but not others" (Broadbent 2013: 158). This objection to risk factor thinking is very different from Krieger's critique of risk factors, first articulated in 1994 (Krieger 1994). Her frustration with causal diagrams featuring web-style representations (a disease/effect surrounded by boxes and lines of risk factors/causes contributing to it)—is that the rote drawing of these boxes and lines serves to distract us from asking why a given population has its particular set of risk factor boxes. As she later elaborated, we should be asking "why, given the identified constellation of risk factors, would the incidence (or prevalence) differ by social group and change over time" (Krieger 2011: 153)? Keyes and Galea echo and cite Krieger's concerns when they elaborate that the "emphasis on identifying risk factors within a paradigm that hunts for precise causal effects," serves to distract us from asking and answering questions about which causal dynamics matter most in a given context (Keyes and Galea 2016: 89).

There are many particular models and approaches for getting at this question, including the Ecosocial Theory that Krieger developed (Krieger 2011). The point I wish to make here is that we need to ask the (right) questions—we need to investigate the "causes of incidence" (Rose 1985). So, contra Broadbent, I agree with Krieger that the problem with risk factor thinking is not that such thinking eschews the Contrastive Model-type discovery of the causes that are jointly sufficient to cause a disease or the particular characteristic cause(s) of the disease; the problem is that risk factor thinking can make us forget that risk factors are variable and malleable. Krieger—one of the co-founders of the Spirit of 1848 Caucus—covertly paraphrases Virchow by saying that one way to improve our causal understanding is to think about the two spiders that each play roles in creating cause-and-effect strands in the web of causation: "one social, one biologic" (Krieger 1994: 896). A desire to defend epidemiological attention to cause of incidence questions is one of the reasons I am writing this book and this chapter about setting appropriate priorities in how we theorize and respond to the causes of population health.

Next, turning to Geoffrey Rose's distinction between "causes of cases" vs. "causes of incidence" can help to pinpoint how Broadbent's philosophy of disease concepts and health causation serves as a tool for investigating the former types of causes, but not the latter. That is, Broadbent and Henle seek to uncover the mechanisms that lead an individual patient to fall ill while their neighbor is well (Exposure to a bacterium? Clogged arteries?), while I agree with Rose and subsequent population health science scholars that we should instead prioritize uncovering the causes that lead one population to have high rates of a given disease, while another population has low rates (Overcrowded housing? Inability to afford a balanced diet?).

Turning attention from "causes of cases" to "causes of incidence"

Two of Geoffrey Rose's foremost contributions to epidemiological theory and to the foundation of population health science were to make two simple distinctions: the "high-risk strategy" vs. the "population strategy" and the "causes of cases" vs. the "causes of incidence" (Rose 1985, 1992). The former distinction—between interventions that target high-risk subpopulations for focused attention vs. interventions that target the entire population—will be discussed at length in Chapter 6. Here, the distinction is between two types of causal explanation for two different types of causal phenomena. As Rose puts it,

> "Why do some individuals have hypertension?" is a quite different question from "Why do some populations have much hypertension, whilst in others it is rare?"
>
> (Rose 1985: 33)

The first question asks why individual patients fall ill, and directs us to search for the set of pathological mechanisms that distinguish sick patients from healthy patients: the "causes of cases" (Rose 1985). The second question asks why some populations' members get ill more often than other populations', and directs us to search for the set of population-level mechanisms that distinguish disease-prone populations from healthier populations: the "causes of incidence" (Rose 1985). For instance, genetic variations make individual people a substantially higher or lower risk of hypertension (Padmanabhan et al. 2015), but these individual-level variations seem to make no causal contribution to the extensively studied massive disparity in hypertension rates between US White and Black populations (Kaufman et al. 2015). Genetics may explain much about sick individuals (causes of cases) but do little to explain why some populations are plagued by hypertension more than other populations (causes of incidence) (Valles 2016b).

Rose's distinction merits some philosophical unpacking. As I argued in two previous papers, these sorts of distinctions—what exactly we are trying to solve with this explanation—are enormously consequential; the important nuances can stretch throughout the entire explanation process, starting with "phenomenon choice" (Valles 2010, 2016a). That work shows how scientists can unknowingly end up in disputes over how to explain something because they had started out by choosing subtly different phenomena to explain. Building upon work by Bromberger and van Fraassen, I argue that we can understand the complexities of competing types of explanations as part of the logic of "why-questions"—what it means to ask why in science (Bromberger 1966; van Fraassen 1990). Van Fraassen explains that when we ask "why?" we are really asking why is the world like this as opposed to some other range of states that the world could be in, the "contrast class" of alternatives. But it is essential to understand that contexts, purposes, goals, and other pragmatic considerations are what determines the proper contrast classes (van Fraassen 1990: 129). The two steps are: first, I decide on a phenomenon to explain based on what I think merits my attention; second, I formulate a why-question in the form of "Why is phenomenon X happening, as opposed to [set of alternative phenomena]" and along the way I should and do have the freedom to choose that set of alternatives based on pragmatic considerations (Valles 2016a).

In this light, we can read (Rose 1985) as delineating a key distinction between two kinds of questions, distinguished by two different sets of contrast classes and associated explanatory goals guiding how we ask and answer the question "why do people get hypertension?":

- Phenomenon 1: some individuals get hypertension and others don't.

  - Why-Question (1) Why do some people get diagnosed with hypertension?
  - Contrast Class 1: … as opposed to having lower blood pressures?

    - Associated research direction: Identify the causes of between-individual variance.
    - For example, identify more of the handful of genes that "in aggregate explain 5%–9% of inter-individual variance in BP" (Huan et al. 2015: 2).

- Phenomenon 2: hypertension incidence varies enormously from population to population.

  - Why-Question (2) Why do some populations have high rates of hypertension diagnoses?
  - Contrast class: … as opposed to having lower rates, like some other populations

    - Associated research direction: Identify the causes of between-population variance.
    - For example, identify more of the environmental causes that make some countries have higher rates than others, for example, lead-glazed pottery used for food service in some countries (Landrigan et al. 2017).

Option 1 above, investigates Rose's "causes of cases" while the second option investigates his "causes of incidence" (Rose 1985).

Rose's work radically challenged epidemiology by directing epidemiologists to devote more attention to the distinct contrast classes and corresponding explanations that are generated when we ask not what separates the "population" of sick people from the "population" of healthy people, but rather what distinguishes the populations in which people tend to get sick from the populations in which people tend to be healthy. It is no coincidence that two of the foundational texts of population health science are Rose's 1992 book elaborating on a 1985 article aptly named "Sick Individuals and Sick Populations" (Rose 1985, 1992), and an edited volume with the even more on-the-nose title, *Why Are Some People Healthy and Others Not?: The Determinants of Health of Populations* (Evans et al. 1994) (see Chapter 2). That legacy continues; Keyes and Galea devote an entire chapter of their book *Population Health Science* to "The Causes of Cases Versus Causes of Incidence" (Keyes and Galea 2016: 25).

Broadbent's book also makes use of the contrast class model of why-questions and explanation, but omits the why-question elaborations added by van Fraassen's work and my work (van Fraassen 1990; Valles 2016a; Broadbent

2013: 72, 100–102). This leaves out the pragmatic flexibility of the choice of contrast class and the consequences of that flexibility.

> While it would be nice to say what characterizes the members of [the contrast class], that must probably be left open. It is a properly scientific question, not a philosophical one, about which possibilities are live ones and which are not from the perspective of best current scientific knowledge.
>
> (Broadbent 2013: 72)

Existing scientific knowledge should indeed constrain which hypothetical states of the world we contrast against what we have observed in the world—for example, we should use the best available data to define what qualifies as a healthy blood pressure range when we ask what makes a patient's blood pressure rise from that range to the hypertensive level. But the existing body of scientific evidence cannot choose between multiple sets of viable contrast classes; scientists must make those choices based on pragmatic considerations. We are forced to make difficult judgments about which scientific questions to ask, and which types of explanation to pursue. Broadbent has built his approach around explaining causes of cases; I am building my account around explaining causes of incidence since I think it is the more promising option for real world health promotion.

Following Rose's advice to attend to the "causes of incidence" is not only a necessary step toward distinct population thinking—attending to "sick populations" rather than aggregates of "sick individuals" (Rose 1985); it is also a necessary step toward promoting health equity. In a 2001 commentary, Weed reminds readers that Rose openly advertised that his advocacy for causes of incidence was radical, all the more so because of "Rose's assertion that our priority should *always* (his word, my emphasis) be the discovery of causes of incidence" and "individual susceptibility will 'cease to matter' if the underlying causes of incidence are removed" (Weed 2001: 440). Ebrahim and Lau's companion commentary helps to understand why this radicalism advances health equity by explaining the significance of "causes of incidence" for the "developing world" (Ebrahim and Lau 2001). They explain how health promotion efforts had long repeated the error of looking for "magic bullet" solutions rooted in causes-of-cases sorts of thinking, such as this line of thought: cases of xerophthalmia (a progressive eye disease) are caused by vitamin A deficiency due to malnutrition; but, vitamin A can be administered with oral supplements; therefore, let's solve xerophthalmia by distributing vitamin supplements to the developing world (Ebrahim and Lau 2001)! Despite many such attempts at magic bullet solutions, malnutrition and other population health problems continued because vitamin supplements do nothing to address the social determinants of nutritional deficiencies, including "poverty," "maternal education," and the "cultural values" that influence poverty and maternal education, and hence influence the foods and supplements that people choose to consume (Ebrahim and Lau 2001: 433). Lack of vitamin A in the diet is a cause of cases, but it leads to folly if we take it to dictate interventions for addressing problems better understood by investigating the causes of incidence. To repeat the passage appearing at the beginning of the chapter:

> A focus only on indicators of health "within the skin" has the disadvantage that upstream interventions tend to be ignored as lying outside the health domain, consigning population health research to remaining at the level of describing *what* but not analyzing *why*.
>
> (McDowell et al. 2004: 391).

Understanding what xerophthalmia's pathogenic mechanisms are does not tell us *why* xerophthalmia and vitamin A deficiency often afflict poor populations but rarely rich ones. Vitamin A pills can at best treat one of the diseases of deprivation, provided we can even get the right doses to the right children at the right times. If we want a permanent and effective solution, we need to look at the upstream causes of vitamin deficiency, including fundamental causes—(lack of) wealth and (lack of) education.

Philosophy of salutogenesis vs. philosophy of pathogenesis

The history of population health science has a curiously complex relationship with the concept "salutogenesis"—*health* causation, used as a sharp contrast with health sciences' long-standing focus on *disease* causation. The concept has been used in both a broad sense and a narrow sense. Broadly, it means what its etymology suggests—an interest in the origins of health, as opposed to the origins of disease. The narrower sense is a more complex model of health and health promotion initially offered by the medical sociologist Aaron Antonovsky (Mittelmark et al. 2017). The Ottawa Charter (Chapter 2 argues it is a linchpin document in establishing health as ethically inseparable from social empowerment) was influenced by salutogenesis (Mcqueen and De Salazar 2011; Eriksson and Lindström 2008). In Fundamental Cause Theory literature, Link and Phelan cite Antonovsky's empirical work, but not Salutogenesis Theory, even though Fundamental Cause Theory and Salutogenesis Theory are likeminded in their interests in the social resources that make health possible (Eriksson and Lindström 2008; Link and Phelan 1995). Keyes and Galea's Population Health Science echoes salutogenesis's view that health is a continuous rather than a discrete phenomenon, but makes no mention of salutogenesis (Keyes and Galea 2016).

Addressing the tension between salutogenesis vs. pathogenesis can help us to address the chapter's earlier question about how to move forward from the aimless listing or diagramming of risk factors. In a 1994 commentary on the Leeds Declaration, an early document in the development of population health science, the editors of *The Lancet* agree with Broadbent's concern regarding the "exaggerated focus on risk factors," but go in a different direction by recommending that we look beyond unitary cause–effect relationships; for example, we should ask "what diets are least likely to cause disease rather than how cholesterol affects the heart" (The Lancet Editors 1994: 429). Hertzman et al., in a chapter for the volume *Why Are Some People Healthy and Others Not?* independently made a similar point that same year—attacking the practice of "disease-based epidemiology" (Hertzman et al. 1994: 81).

Hertzman et al.'s objection to "disease-based epidemiology" is tied to a variant of life course thinking, the concept I endorse in Chapter 3 and incorporate into my definition of health. As the authors explain, individual diseases, even causes of death, are often so distant from the site of the real action (so to speak) that data such as rates of influenza death in the elderly "are frequently unworthy of analysis" (Hertzman et al. 1994: 82). Pointing to influenza as the proximate cause is correct, but proximate causes are superficial if health's causes and effects develop over an entire lifespan. So, a proximate cause of death, such as a case of the flu, is obviously important to the patients (it is their cause of death!), but is minimally informative to population health scientists who wish to understand and promote healthy lives. The flu is simply the metaphorical "straw that broke the camel's back." One's vulnerability to influenza infections and the corresponding morbidity and mortality, is built up over a lifetime through: a diet that is/isn't conducive to immune system health, accumulated exposure to second-hand smoke and other airborne particulates, the level of income and associated ability to access healthcare services such as up-to-date influenza vaccines, and so on. These prior causes—some directly traceable to fundamental causes such as wealth—together shape the health trajectory of a person's life, including how likely a person is to be infected by the flu while elderly, and how likely they are to die from that infection. No matter what, the fact that an elderly patient died of the flu tells us little about how to promote overall health in the elderly and in those who are not yet elderly. The problem remains in contemporary global public health data. The Global Burden of Disease Study is a massive and influential international health-monitoring program. But, since most mental illnesses, including depression, do not appear as causes of death on death certificates, the study has estimated that "mental disorders appear to only account for 0.5% of total years of life lost," though if one looks at the underlying causes of deaths, it appears that "14.3% of deaths worldwide … are attributable to mental disorders" (Vigo et al. 2016: 174).

As the Leeds Declaration puts it, "there is an urgent need to re-focus upstream, to move away from focusing predominantly on individual risks towards the social structures and processes within which health originates" (The Lancet Editors 1994: 431). It's not just single disease-based epidemiology that needs its preeminence challenged, it's the even more basic assumption that we should direct our attention to disease rather than to health (The Lancet Editors 1994). The influential US National Association of County & City Health Officials extended this objection to institutional structures by arguing:

> organizing health department programs around single diseases, risk factors, and populations made it difficult to consider the broad spectrum of poor

health associated with deeper social inequalities or to forge a practice that could more directly address the sources of health inequities.

(National Association of County & City Health Officials 2014: 1)

More recently, the textbook *Population Health* echoes the "upstream" term in the title of its concluding chapter, and argues, "we also have learned that health is a complex system and that the 'medical reductionism' solution, such as single disease management, is not going to solve our population health concerns" (Edington and Schultz 2011).

In light of the above, I read Broadbent's approach to epidemiology as effect-ively doubling down on the strategy of focusing on disease/pathogenesis, not least because applying his Contrastive Model of Disease would lead to the creat-ing of many more new diseases. For instance:

lung cancer could no longer be regarded as a disease if we came to know conclusively that no common aetiology for all cases existed. It would be a grouping of symptoms, perhaps caused by a number of other diseases, each with a distinctive aetiology.

(Broadbent 2013: 160)

In her review of his book, Plutynski points out that the Contrastive Model threatens to create an explosion of new diseases exclusively on the basis of etiology, regard-less of the, also important, considerations like how diseases are similar or different in their prognosis or their treatments: "diseases will multiply beyond manageabil-ity, given that many diseases have so many distinctive causes (cancers alone will number not in the hundreds, but perhaps in the hundreds of thousands)" (Plutynski 2014: 110). What is the payoff for this move? Broadbent wishes to reject multifac-torial thinking, which "provides no way of discriminating between a flower and a weed," in the meadow of causes. Broadbent is able to solve the problem of an unmanageable proliferation of causes (too many risk factors!) only by opting for an unmanageable proliferation of effects (too many diseases!). I share the desire to find some amount of order—and the potential for intervening thereupon—in the chaos of population-level health causation. I disagree about how to do so.

Conclusion

This chapter is framed in part as a contrast between my views on health causa-tion and Broadbent's. Different health causation concepts and philosophies each serve some priorities and goals better than others. My objection to Broadbent's approach to disease concepts and causation is that it serves the goal of uncover-ing the causes of (individual) cases, and ill serves the goal of uncovering the causes of (diverging population) incidence. This is a problem because, as I have argued, the causes of incidence are a more pressing and more promising line of research for those who wish to improve the health of populations, especially the most needy populations.

In this chapter, I advocate for the importance of investigating and intervening in upstream causes. I do not argue that more proximate causes, or mechanisms, are unimportant. And, unlike Krieger, I do not think that advocates of upstream health research and interventions (e.g., Fundamental Cause Theory) have excessively pitted upstream vs. downstream causes (distal vs. proximate) against each other. Krieger worries that such a dichotomization serves to conceal the real dynamics at work: "levels" (an individual person, an institution, etc.), "pathways" (trajectories of development, causal mechanisms of social structure on individual health, etc.) and "power" (social relations, such as gender roles, constraining individuals' and populations' possibilities) (Krieger 2008: 228). On this point, I agree more with Freese and Lutfey, who see Fundamental Cause Theory as a complement to other work in population health science. Krieger's Ecosocial Theory happens to be an especially comprehensive and promising contribution to that body of work (Krieger appears often in this book). In an article co-authored with epidemiologist colleagues, Broadbent and his co-authors phrased it well when they called for epidemiologists to adopt "a pragmatic pluralism about concepts of causality" (Vandenbroucke et al. 2016: 1784). Freese and Lutfey elaborate that a properly "incisive" explanation of proximate causes/mechanisms:

> makes sense of a diverse set of mechanisms, offers predictive insight into why the population distribution of disease will be surprisingly robust to changes in the causes of ill-health, and calls attention to the possibility of more encompassing interventions.
>
> (Freese and Lutfey 2011: 69)

And therein is the rationale for why fundamental causes merit special attention even though both they and more proximate causes are all important: fundamental causes help direct us to understand why many interventions on proximate interventions fail, and guide us to more wide-ranging and effective interventions. As Ebrahim and Lau highlight in their critique of "magic bullet" solutions, diet-related vitamin deficiency is a measurable and urgent population health problem, but this does not necessarily mean that handing out more vitamins is the best solution (Ebrahim and Lau 2001).

Fundamental causes are flexible features of social life that predictably generate positive or negative health effects, through flexible and unpredictable mechanisms and specific health outcomes. It is a matter of historical inevitability that new infectious diseases will sporadically emerge, and the world will soon contend with the next SARS, MERS, strain of influenza, etc. When some groundbreaking new medication arrives, it will first benefit those with more status and resources—those who have the benefit of flexible social buffers such as prestige, money, racial privilege, and an absence of stigma against them. Recall that during the 2014 Ebola outbreak in West Africa, it was two White medical missionaries—rather than the thousands of local patients—who had the opportunity to receive a promising experimental treatment (Schuklenk 2014).

Missteps in how we approach causation in health promotion lead to problems in the implementation of responses. Such missteps have impeded many of the global AIDS responses, each of which struggle with unique milieus of social dynamics of sexuality, class, immigration status, social stigma, etc. Before ending this chapter, it is worth noting here that Link and Phelan's classic paper not only uses HIV as one example of their aforementioned theoretical points about population health causation, but it also correctly predicted that HIV's growing prevalence in low SES brackets would exacerbate inequalities between populations (Link and Phelan 1995). This brings us to the chapter's case study of the Brazil's HIV/AIDS response, which illustrates the promises and pitfalls of certain theories and practices of population health science causation.

Case study: Brazil's AIDS response

Brazil is famous for declaring that HIV antiretroviral drugs (Highly Active Antiretroviral Therapy—HAART—which both ameliorate the immunosuppression effects of HIV and reduce transmission risk) are a human right, and building a surprisingly effective program to honor that right for its citizens (Nunn 2009). In the process, the country shocked the world by committing to a 15-year trade battle against the US and the global pharmaceutical industry over the intellectual property rights for HAART drugs, which restricted the affordable production and distribution of the drugs (Nunn 2009). The story is complex, but Brazil's response has been widely lauded for exceeding expectations given the limited resources and abundant obstacles. Its successes, and failures, help to illustrate this chapter's arguments about which population health causes to prioritize, and why.

Through the lens of Fundamental Cause Theory, Brazil's guarantee of universal HAART, the cornerstone of HIV/AIDS clinical care, weakened the causal path between (lack of) money and (in)ability to obtain HIV treatment. This is an outstanding accomplishment for public health and human rights (Taket 2012). Though, as the Black Report famously found in the UK (see Chapter 2), a government guarantee of universal medical care does not automatically mean that the needy will fully benefit from these nominally available resources, nor does universal healthcare address the many determinants of health that lay largely out of the reach of healthcare institutions (Black et al. 1980). Fundamental Cause Theory warns that erasing one pathway from a fundamental cause to an outcome can still leave other pathways between them in place (Phelan and Link 2015; Hatzenbuehler et al. 2013). And indeed, it turned out that factors such as wait times at government clinics and transportation costs continue to impede some Brazilians in need from receiving the guaranteed HAART (Hoffmann et al. 2016).

Stigma is a particularly powerful fundamental cause affecting HIV/AIDS. Empirical work also finds that HIV stigma in Brazil reinforces existing social inequities by most potently afflicting HIV+ members of populations that are already marginalized—the "poor, those with lower education, sex workers and people with a history of drug use" (Kerrigan et al. 2017). To combat stigma surrounding condom use, Brazil's government has been pursuing efforts such as promoting public campaigns to normalize condom use, especially among young people (Coelho 2016). Figure 5.1 gives an example of a government public education effort designed for the 2017 Carnival celebrations, depicting revelers proudly holding condoms in the air. Government HIV/AIDS efforts in Brazil have long embraced close relationships with civil society, which facilitates addressing fundamental causes rooted in everyday life. Acting boldly, "AIDS officials in fact proactively sought out partnerships to work with AIDS and gay NGOs, conservative church leaders, and even the sex pornography industry to provide care and treatment" (Gómez 2016). Even as the clout of the evangelical Christian community has increased, the Government has actively resisted direct and indirect attempts to shift the AIDS response to manifest a more politically and religiously conservative moral disapproval of gay Brazilians and Brazilians in the sex work industry (Gómez 2016).

It is important to remember that Brazil is a former colony of Portugal, and its population health efforts occur against the backdrop of colonial power dynamics, issues previously raised in the case studies in Chapters 2 (the Standing Rock Sioux) and 3 (Aboriginal Australians). One way this complicates the Brazil case is that former President Cardoso reports that he began the reform of the AIDS response partly as a means of achieving a broader goal: building the prestige ("reputation") of Brazil as a whole (Gómez 2010). Prestige is indeed one of the

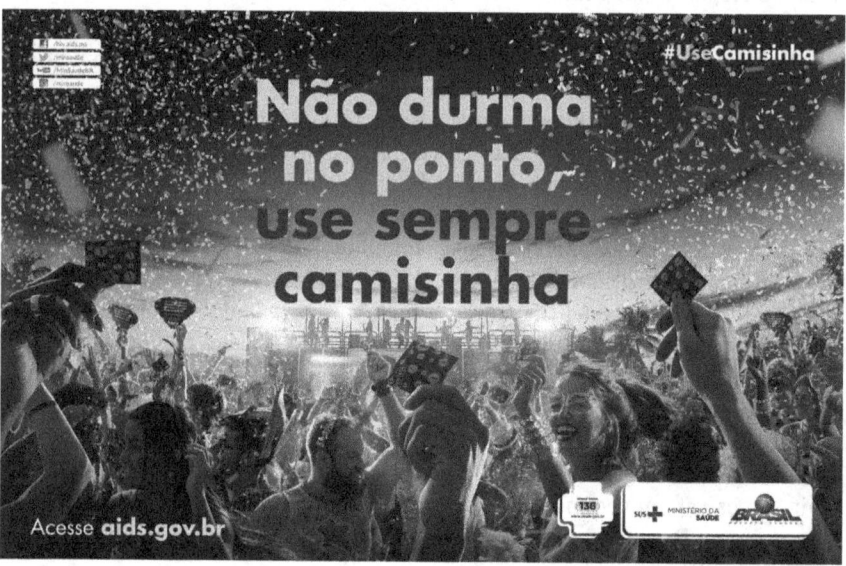

Figure 5.1 "Não durma no ponto, use sempre camisinha" (idiomatic, roughly "don't fall asleep at the switch, always use a condom"). A government advertisement promoting condom use.

Source: www.aids.gov.br/sites/default/files/campanhas/2017/64557/ms_carnaval_abrigo_onibus.pdf.

fundamental causes of health cited by Link and Phelan (1995). In one reading, Brazil's AIDS strategy pursued a suite of interventions to address fundamental causes of health in order to manage its AIDS epidemic, which in turn was part of a larger strategy to grow its prestige. Brazil's rising prestige (e.g., as one of the so-called BRIC countries with increasing political and economic clout) probably served it well during a 2016 global campaign in the months preceding the Rio Olympics, which strove to delay, cancel or relocate them for fear of spreading Zika globally (Belluck 2016). The effort failed, Brazil averted a potentially very damaging economic loss from a disruption of the games and no infections were recorded among the Olympic attendees (World Health Organization 2016b). The health of a population both affects, and is affected by, its prestige.

AIDS is one of the most poignant illustrations of the ways that risk factor thinking can go awry, both ethically and empirically. For example, the pervasive representation of homosexuality as a risk factor for AIDS in men is both an ethical failure and an epistemic failure: it is stigmatizing and misleading (Katikireddi and Valles 2015). It is true that gay men have relatively high rates of AIDS in many populations. But to treat gayness as a risk factor conflates sexual orientation (e.g., being a man who is primarily sexually attracted to men, regardless of sexual behaviors) and sexual status/behavior (e.g., being a man who has sex with men, regardless of sexual orientation) (van Anders 2015). And, even a putative risk factor such as male–male sex serves to conceal the enormous variability of riskiness between different sexual practices (e.g., the risk of HIV transmission via oral sex is vanishingly small) (Patel et al. 2014).

To repeat Krieger's guiding questions from above, it is imperative to ask, "why, given the identified constellation of risk factors, would the incidence (or prevalence) differ by social group and change over time" (Krieger 2011: 153).[3] And we all must ask this, not just population health scientists. If it is in some sense an HIV risk factor for a man to have sex with another man, we must inter-rogate why this is the case, and act accordingly. We must interrogate the role of homophobia in Brazil—and elsewhere—in keeping same-sex couples from having socially sanctioned long-term relationships (when this is something they wish to have) (Costa et al. 2013). We must also interrogate the historical contin-gencies of the history of AIDS as initially a disease of gay men and then other marginalized populations such as users of illicit injection drugs, leading to a legacy of high HIV rates in the associated communities such that transmission is more likely just by virtue of the fact that relatively more of their peers are HIV+ (even aside from any specific risky behaviors, such as needle sharing).

Knowledge about "causes of cases" can only take us so far. By the end of the 1980s, HIV had been isolated and identified as the cause of AIDS; transmission by needle sharing, vaginal sex and anal sex had been established; condoms had been identified as a prophylaxis; and antiretroviral drugs had begun reaching the market (Harden 2012). Knowledge about the causes of cases continues to guide the development of improved drugs and perhaps even a vaccine and/or a total ("sterilizing") cure. In the meantime, Brazil's populations and other populations across the world have shown the enduring power of fundamental causes of health other than money to affect HIV/AIDS population health. As one of the largest countries in the world, and an especially culturally/ethnically diverse one at that, it faced the daunting challenge of being afflicted by a stigmatized disease that attacks under-resourced countries, and which had variable incidence within the country's expansive geography. Brazil's ingenious solution to the problem was to strike a balance between accountability and human rights guarantees at the national level with a policy of decentralization, through which local AIDS governance functions were handed out to local governments to tailor to their own needs (Berkman et al. 2005; Gómez 2010). The social dynamics and health governance needs of São Paulo urbanites are not the same as the social dynamics and health governance needs of rural farmers. Chapter 7 will continue the discussion of health governance and the philosophy thereof.

HIV raised unusual issues in salutogenesis and pathogenesis partly because it is a discrete virus, yet causes a plethora of health harms due to its effect of suppressing the immune system. It is not readily subjected to the sort of disease-based epidemiology decried by Hertzman et al. (Hertzman et al. 1994: 81). It is abundantly obvious that addressing HIV/AIDS necessitates addressing the other diseases it causes though suppressing the immune system. In Brazil the salutogenesis vs. pathogenesis tension—the focus on health vs. disease—is more complicated. Brazil happened to be in a particularly good position to philosophically appreciate the significance of these sorts of issues because of the influence of social medicine advocates who had taken up positions in Brazil's health governance institutions (Nunn 2009: 31–34). As discussed in Chapter 2, South America's social medicine scholars and activists (Chile's President, Salvador Allende is the most famous) took inspiration from theorists such as Virchow and Engels (part of the intellectual camp targeted by Henle) to carry on the philosophical commitment to jointly promoting anti-colonialism, social justice, health equity and overall population well-being (Diez Roux 2016; Labonté et al. 2005; Krieger and Birn 1998; Waitzkin 2007). The philosophy of Latin American social medicine already incorporated concepts such as health causation as a dynamic social process, social conditions as health causes, and health as the positive presence of social well-being (Waitzkin 2007). As in the Chapter 2 and 3 case studies—the Standing Rock Sioux's understanding of health as social, and Aboriginal Australians' understanding of health as a phenomenon extended over the life course—populations living in the legacy of colonial repression understood health and well-being in ways that US-Canada-Europe-dominated population health science needed to gradually catch up to.

From here we now turn to matters of population health methodology. Health equity is a central goal of population health science, and the upcoming Chapter 6 discussion of equity-minded population health methodological trade-offs will lead directly to Chapter 7's more general analysis of health equity in population health science.

Notes

1 Full disclosure: I am a member of the caucus.
2 For a fuller history, see Hamlin (1998).
3 "Incidence" refers to the rate of new cases of a condition in a population over a period of time, while "prevalence" refers to the total proportion of a population with the condition at a given time.

Works cited

Belluck, P. (2016) WHO issues Zika warnings for Rio travel, but resists calls to delay games. *New York Times*. New York: New York Times Company, B8.

Berkman, A., Garcia, J., Muñoz-Laboy, M., et al. (2005) A critical analysis of the Brazilian response to HIV/AIDS: Lessons learned for controlling and mitigating the epidemic in developing countries. *American Journal of Public Health* 95, 1162–1172.

Birn, A.-E. (2009) Making it politic(al): Closing the gap in a generation: Health equity through action on the social determinants of health. *Social Medicine* 4, 166–182.

Black, D., Morris, J., Smith, C. and Townsend, P. (1980) Inequalities in Health: Report of a Research Working Group on Inequalities in Health. London: Department of Health and Social Security.

Broadbent, A. (2013) *Philosophy of Epidemiology*. New York: Palgrave Macmillan.

Broadbent, A. (2014) Disease as a theoretical concept: The case of "HPV-itis." *Studies in History and Philosophy of Biological and Biomedical Sciences* 48, 250–257.

Bromberger, S. (1966) Why-Questions. In: Colodny, R. G. (ed.) *Mind and Cosmos: Essays in Contemporary Science and Philosophy*. Pittsburgh: University of Pittsburgh Press, 86–111.

Carter, K. C. (2003) *The Rise of Causal Concepts of Disease: Case Histories*. Aldershot: Ashgate.

Chetty, R., Stepner, M., Abraham, S., et al. (2016) The association between income and life expectancy in the United States, 2001–2014. *Journal of the American Medical Association* 315, 1750–1766.

Coelho, N. (2016) Brazil breaks the record of people undergoing treatment against HIV and AIDS. STD, AIDS and Viral Hepatitis Department. Press release. Agência Saúde Press Service, Brasilia, Brazil.

Costa, A. B., Peroni, R. O., Bandeira, D. R. and Nardi, H. C. (2013) Homophobia or sexism? A systematic review of prejudice against nonheterosexual orientation in Brazil. *International Journal of Psychology* 48, 900–909.

Dammann, O. (2015) Epidemiological explanations. *Philosophy of Science* 82, 509–519.

Diez Roux, A. V. (2016) On the distinction—or lack of distinction—between population health and public health. *American Journal of Public Health* 106, 619–620.

Doku, D. T. and Neupane, S. (2015) Double burden of malnutrition: Increasing overweight and obesity and stall underweight trends among Ghanaian women. *BMC Public Health* 15, 670.

Dowdy, D. W. and Pai, M. (2012) Bridging the gap between knowledge and health: The epidemiologist as accountable health advocate ("AHA!"). *Epidemiology* 23, 914–918.

Ebrahim, S. and Lau, E. (2001) Commentary: Sick populations and sick individuals. *International Journal of Epidemiology* 30, 433–434.

Edington, D. W. and Schultz, A. B. (2011) The Future of Population Health: Moving Upstream. In: Nash, D. B., Reifsnyder, J., Fabius, R. J., et al. (eds) *Population Health: Creating a Culture of Wellness.* Sudbury, MA: Jones & Bartlett Publishers.

Eriksson, M. and Lindström, B. (2008) A salutogenic interpretation of the Ottawa Charter. *Health Promotion International* 23, 190–199.

Evans, R. G., Barer, M. L. and Marmor, T. R. (1994) *Why Are Some People Healthy and Others Not? The Determinants of Health of Populations.* New York: Aldine De Gruyter.

Freese, J. and Lutfey, K. (2011) Fundamental Causality: Challenges of an Animating Concept for Medical Sociology. In: Pescosolido, B. A., Martin, J. K., McLeod, J. D., et al. (eds) *Handbook of the Sociology of Health, Illness, and Healing.* New York: Springer, 67–81.

Galea, S. (2018) *Healthier: Fifty Thoughts on the Foundations of Population Health.* New York: Oxford University Presss.

Gómez, E. J. (2010) What the United States can learn from Brazil in response to HIV/AIDS: International reputation and strategic centralization in a context of health policy devolution. *Health Policy and Planning* 25, 529–541.

Gómez, E. J. (2016) Crafting AIDS policy in Brazil and Russia: State-civil societal ties, institutionalised morals, and foreign policy aspiration. *Global Public Health* 11, 1148–1168.

Hamlin, C. (1998) *Public Health and Social Justice in the Age of Chadwick: Britain, 1800–1854.* Cambridga: Cambridge University Press.

Harden, V. A. (2012) *AIDS at 30: A History.* Washington, DC: Potomac Books, Inc.

Hatzenbuehler, M. L., Phelan, J. C. and Link, B. G. (2013) Stigma as a fundamental cause of population health inequalities. *American Journal of Public Health* 103, 813–821.

Hertzman, C., Frank, J. and Evans, R. G. (1994) Heterogeneities in Health Status and the Determinants of Population Health. In: Evans, R. G., Barer, M. L. and Marmor, T. R. (eds) *Why Are Some People Healthy and Others Not?* New York: Aldine De Gruyter.

Hill, A. B. (1965) The environment and disease: Association or causation? *Proceedings of the Royal Society of Medicine* 58, 295–300.

Hoffmann, M., MacCarthy, S., Batson, A., et al. (2016) Barriers along the care cascade of HIV-infected men in a large urban center of Brazil. *AIDS Care* 28, 57–62.

Huan, T., Esko, T., Peters, M. J., et al. (2015) A meta-analysis of gene expression signatures of blood pressure and hypertension. *PLOS Genetics* 11, e1005035.

Jones, C. P., Jones, C. Y., Perry, G. S., et al. (2009) Addressing the social determinants of children's health: A cliff analogy. *Journal of Health Care for the Poor and Underserved* 20, 1–12.

Katikireddi, S. V. and Valles, S. A. (2015) Coupled ethical-epistemic analysis of public health research and practice: Categorizing variables to improve population health and equity. *American Journal of Public Health* 105, e36–e42.

Kaufman, J. S., Dolman, L., Rushani, D. and Cooper, R. S. (2015) The contribution of genomic research to explaining racial disparities in cardiovascular disease: A systematic review. *American Journal of Epidemiology* 181, 464–472.

Kerrigan, D., Vazzano, A., Bertoni, N., et al. (2017) Stigma, discrimination and HIV outcomes among people living with HIV in Rio de Janeiro, Brazil: The intersection of multiple social inequalities. *Global Public Health* 12, 185–199.

Keyes, K. M. and Galea, S. (2016) *Population Health Science.* New York: Oxford University Press.

Krieger, N. (1994) Epidemiology and the web of causation: Has anyone seen the spider? *Social Science & Medicine* 39, 887–903.

Krieger, N. (2008) Proximal, distal, and the politics of causation: What's level got to do with it? *American Journal of Public Health* 98, 221–230.

Krieger, N. (2011) *Epidemiology and the People's Health: Theory and Context.* New York: Oxford University Press.

Krieger, N. and Birn, A.-E. (1998) A vision of social justice as the foundation of public health: Commemorating 150 years of the spirit of 1848. *American Journal of Public Health* 88, 1603–1606.

Labonté, R., Polanyi, M., Muhajarine, N., et al. (2005) Beyond the divides: Towards critical population health research. *Critical Public Health* 15, 5–17.

Landrigan, P. J., Fuller, R., Acosta, N. J. R., et al. (2017) The Lancet Commission on pollution and health. *The Lancet.*

Link, B. G. and Phelan, J. (1995) Social conditions as fundamental causes of disease. *Journal of Health and Social Behavior* 35, 80–94.

Manyanga, T., El-Sayed, H., Doku, D. T. and Randall, J. R. (2014) The prevalence of underweight, overweight, obesity and associated risk factors among school-going adolescents in seven African countries. *BMC Public Health* 14, 1.

Marmot, M. (2004) *The Status Syndrome: How Social Standing Affects Our Health and Longevity.* New York: Henry Holt and Company.

Marmot, M. G., Shipley, M. J. and Rose, G. (1984) Inequalities in death—specific explanations of a general pattern? *The Lancet* 323, 1003–1006.

McDowell, I., Spasoff, R. A. and Kristjansson, B. (2004) On the classification of population health measurements. *American Journal of Public Health* 94, 388–393.

McQueen, D. V. and De Salazar, L. (2011) Health promotion, the Ottawa Charter and "developing personal skills": A compact history of 25 years. *Health Promotion International* 26, ii194-ii201.

Mittelmark, M. B., Sagy, S., Eriksson, M., et al. (2017) *The Handbook of Salutogenesis.* Cham, Switzerland: Springer.

Montez, J. K., Zajacova, A. and Hayward, M. D. (2017) Contextualizing the social determinants of health: Disparities in disability by educational attainment across US states. *American Journal of Public Health* 107, 1101–1108.

National Association of County & City Health Officials. (2014) Expanding the Boundaries: Health Equity and Public Health Practice. Washington, DC: National Association of County & City Health Officials.

Nguyen, B. T., Shuval, K., Bertmann, F. and Yaroch, A. L. (2015) The Supplemental Nutrition Assistance Program, food insecurity, dietary quality, and obesity among US adults. *American Journal of Public Health* 105, 1453–1459.

Nunn, A. (2009) *The Politics and History of AIDS Treatment in Brazil.* New York: Springer Science+Business Media.

Padmanabhan, S., Caulfield, M. and Dominiczak, A. F. (2015) Genetic and molecular aspects of hypertension. *Circulation Research* 116, 937–959.

Paradies, Y., Ben, J., Denson, N., et al. (2015) Racism as a determinant of health: A systematic review and meta-analysis. *PloS One* 10, e0138511.

Patel, P., Borkowf, C. B., Brooks, J. T., et al. (2014) Estimating per-act HIV transmission risk: A systematic review. *Aids* 28, 1509–1519.

Phelan, J. C. and Link, B. G. (2005) Controlling disease and creating disparities: A fundamental cause perspective. *The Journals of Gerontology Series B: Psychological Sciences and Social Sciences* 60, S27–S33.

Phelan, J. C. and Link, B. G. (2015) Is racism a fundamental cause of inequalities in health? *Annual Review of Sociology* 41, 311–330.

Phelan, J. C., Link, B. G. and Tehranifar, P. (2010) Social conditions as fundamental causes of health inequalities: Theory, evidence, and policy implications. *Journal of Health and Social Behavior* 51, S28–S40.

Plutynski, A. (2014) Philosophy of epidemiology. *Studies in History and Philosophy of Biological and Biomedical Sciences* 46, 107–111.

Reich, A. D., Hansen, H. B. and Link, B. G. (2016) Fundamental interventions: How clinicians can address the fundamental causes of disease. *Journal of Bioethical Inquiry* 13, 185–192.

Rose, G. (1985) Sick individuals and sick populations. *International Journal of Epidemiology* 14, 32–38.

Rose, G. (1992) *The Strategy of Preventive Medicine.* New York: Oxford University Press.

Schuklenk, U. (2014) Bioethics and the Ebola outbreak in West Africa. *Developing World Bioethics* 14, ii–iii.

Shea, K. M., Kammerer, J. S., Winston, C. A., et al. (2014) Estimated rate of reactivation of latent tuberculosis infection in the United States, overall and by population subgroup. *American Journal of Epidemiology* 179, 216–225.

Ståhl, T., Wismar, M., Ollila, E., et al. (2006) *Health in All Policies: Prospects and Potentials.* Finland: Finnish Ministry of Social Affairs and Health.

Taket, A. (2012) *Health Equity, Social Justice and Human Rights.* Abingdon: Routledge.

The Lancet Editors. (1994) Population health looking upstream. *The Lancet* 343, 429–432.

Valles, S. A. (2010) The mystery of the mystery of common genetic diseases. *Biology and Philosophy* 25, 183–201.

Valles, S. A. (2016a) The challenges of choosing and explaining a phenomenon in epidemiological research on the "Hispanic Paradox." *Theoretical Medicine and Bioethics* 37, 129–148.

Valles, S. A. (2016b) Race in Medicine. In: Solomon, M., Simon, J. R. and Kincaid, H. (eds) *The Routledge Companion to Philosophy of Medicine.* New York: Routledge, 419–431.

van Anders, S. M. (2015) Beyond sexual orientation: Integrating gender/sex and diverse sexualities via sexual configurations theory. *Archives of Sexual Behavior* 44, 1177–1213.

van Fraassen, B. C. (1990) *The Scientific Image.* New York: Oxford University Press.

Vandenbroucke, J. P., Broadbent, A. and Pearce, N. (2016) Causality and causal inference in epidemiology: The need for a pluralistic approach. *International Journal of Epidemiology* 45, 1776–1786.

Vigo, D., Thornicroft, G. and Atun, R. (2016) Estimating the true global burden of mental illness. *The Lancet Psychiatry* 3, 171–178.

Waitzkin, H. (2007) Political Economic Systems and the Health of Populations: Historical Thought and Current Directions. In: Galea, S. (ed.) *Macrosocial Determinants of Population Health.* New York: Springer Science Business Media, 105–138.

Ward, A. (2007) The social epidemiologic concept of fundamental cause. *Theoretical Medicine and Bioethics* 28, 465–485.

Weed, D. L. (2001) Commentary: A radical future for public health. *International Journal of Epidemiology* 30, 440–441.

Weisberg, M. (2006) Robustness analysis. *Philosophy of Science* 73, 730–742.

Woodward, J. (2010) Causation in biology: Stability, specificity, and the choice of levels of explanation. *Biology & Philosophy* 25, 287–318.

World Health Organization. (2016a) Global Tuberculosis Report 2016. www.who.int/tb/ publications/global_report/en/. Geneva: World Health Organization.

World Health Organization. (2016b) Situation Report: Zika Virus, Microcephaly, Guillain-Barré Syndrome, August 25 2016. Geneva: World Health Organization.

Yadavendu, V. K. (2014) *Shifting Paradigms in Public Health*. New Delhi: Springer India.

Part III

How can population health science better promote health equity?

6 Managing the inevitable trade-offs in population health science practice

Introduction

Chapter 6 comprises the first half of this book's third and final section before Chapter 8's conclusion. The preceding section offered philosophical arguments for how to identify the most important causes in population health science. First, Chapter 4 argued for the need to adopt a broad model of public/population health, looking for potential remediable causes of health in all policies and in all other corners of populations' socioenvironmental contexts: climate change policies, wage laws, workplace environment, etc. Then, Chapter 5 argued for the need to pay attention to the upstream causes of health, especially the so-called "fundamental causes" of health, the flexible social buffers that leave people more or less protected against populations' diverse and shifting health risks. This section picks up the thread by asking how population health science can carry out the goal of promoting equitable health patterns within and among human populations. Population health science is very much concerned with ameliorating these patterns—making them more equitable. Looking ahead to the second half of this section, Chapter 7 will explore how population health science fits within the debates over what health equity is. As in the case of debates over what health is (featured in Chapter 3), I argue that extracting and elaborating on some insights from within the population health science literature can offer a novel perspective on an old question, while also leaving much room for pluralism. But first, this chapter will argue that a set of four central methodological challenges stand in the way of population health as it pursues equity-serving research and interventions. This order in this section—investigating the obstacles to equitable health practices before investigating what equity is in the first place—might seem backward, but as I have repeated throughout this book, the entirety of the population health framework, including the methodological challenges featured in this chapter and even including the nature of its equity concepts, are best understood as evolving reactions to practical empirical findings and the constraints thereon.

This chapter will argue that population health framework efforts toward the goal of health for all requires grappling with two pairs of linked methodological challenges: (1) How should population health researchers balance the benefits and drawbacks of lumping vs. splitting when carving out specific populations to sample during research and when deciding how broadly to make inferences during research? (2) Relatedly, how should population health interventions trade off the relative merits of population health interventions, ones that focus efforts and resources on high-risk populations vs. ones that target the entire population? These two detail-oriented strategic methodological questions must be understood in the context of two larger questions about the direction of the field: (3) How can population health science, which treats population health improvement as its ultimate goal, fruitfully work alongside efforts that are committed to elements of health science that population health science was formed to reject (especially programs that assume the healthcare sector can and should be the center of population health promotion)? (4) How can population health science reconcile the pragmatic needs of its practices with evidence-based medicine's calls to rely more heavily on evidence from strictly controlled experiments, given that such data about social determinants of health and other causes prioritized by population health science are rare and exceptionally difficult to collect? The answers to all of these questions are complex—if they were not so complex they would not merit attention in this chapter. In all four cases, I offer preliminary guidance for how to manage the trade-offs.

The problem of heterogeneity: lumping vs. splitting in population health

Human populations have heterogeneous health experiences, so measurement strategies and interventions must take into account the inevitable heterogeneity. The need to measure/address patterns of variation, and manage the knowledge that not all heterogeneity will indeed get measured/addressed, creates the need to contend with the classic problem shared by all population-level life sciences: lumping vs. splitting. When is it appropriate to group together a heterogeneous group during research/intervention because of their set of similarities, and when is it appropriate to divide them into subgroups in order to acknowledge their differences?

Population health science is deeply committed to equitable health promotion, under an empirical understanding of health as a social and life course phenomenon shaped greatly or even primarily by social and environmental determinants. This section will recommend a pair of criteria as heuristics for helping to resolve lumping vs. splitting conundrums. (1) Drawing on insights from Rose and from Hertzman et al. in their respective works at the founding of contemporary population health science, I advocate for selecting lumps/splits that uncover the causes of between-population health variation ("causes of incidence") (Hertzman et al. 1994; Rose 1985). (2) Adapting a point made by Maglo, I also propose that helping the most needy can function as a tie-breaker during cases of uncertainty in lumping vs. splitting, as a means of recognizing that population health equity compels us to attend to those who would be otherwise marginalized.

The process of lumping things into a small number of groups or splitting them into many groups, famously has no objectively "right" answers (Love 2007). Since before Darwin's time, biologists specializing in systematics have openly struggled with this challenge during their attempts to classify species (Endersby 2009). Biological processes and entities tend to defy unambiguously correct classifications and lumping into broader groupings vs. splitting into a larger number of narrower groupings is driven by a combination of theoretical inclination and individual preference (Love 2007). Applied population health science work requires using imperfect judgment to somehow divide up human variation. Should we err on the side of differentiating between subgroups with many similarities but also some discernible differences, or err on the side of combining together those somewhat different subgroups on the grounds that they are similar enough (Endersby 2009)? If we are too fine-grained in our analyses, we risk losing the ability to detect any statistically meaningful inferences from the data. For example, a study of obesity trends in a city might find value in splitting the data into multiple neighborhoods to see how smaller geographic areas vary due to factors such as differing social/environmental resources. It would probably be unwise to keep splitting until the researchers end up separately analyzing each individual household as a micro-geographic region unto itself. On the other hand, aggregating all of the neighborhoods together and effectively ignoring differences between them, would conceal disparities between the neighborhoods' income levels, access to walking paths and bike lanes, and other factors relevant to obesity trends.

Venkatapuram, in *Health Justice*, points to the lumping vs. splitting problem as a particularly intriguing epistemic challenge: "one of the interesting aspects of population level analysis is the question of where to draw the borders of the population or the place where the health issue is taking place" (Venkatapuram 2011). In population health contexts, he argues, it is easy to forget that even though nations might be effective population groupings to identify and collect data on, they are biologically arbitrary groupings and if we lose sight of their arbitrariness we might start believing that they are automatically the best groupings for carrying out interventions. I have previously illustrated this in a philosophical analysis of research on US Hispanic health, wherein one major obstacle is that health and vital statistics records are collected independently by individual nations (Valles 2016). If a Mexico-born migrant is diagnosed with lung cancer in the US, emigrates back to Mexico, and then dies from the cancer there, then their cancer diagnosis would only be recorded in US statistics but their cancer death would only be recorded in Mexico's statistics, skewing both countries' data on trends in lung cancer mortality. In the case of Hispanic health, the nation-level grouping has led to the perpetuation of a shocking level of uncertainty about the health status of US Hispanics, including the so-called Hispanic Paradox phenomenon, in which Hispanics appear to somehow resist some negative effects of social determinants of health by being healthier than one would expect for a disproportionately poor and marginalized minority population (Valles 2016). The existence of the phenomenon is disputed (it may be a data collection artifact as suggested in the previous example), and if a health benefit effect does exist then its mechanism remains unclear (Valles 2016; Cortes-Bergoderi et al. 2013; Ruiz et al. 2013). And, one of the main reasons for this unresolved status is that "Hispanic" is an exceptionally heterogeneous pan-ethnicity that was only recently formulated and intentionally left vague enough to lump together US-born Chilean Americans, Afro-Cuban immigrants, etc. (Valles 2016).

It is particularly imperative that population health research and interventions be sensitive to known subpopulations with health profiles that are homogeneous enough to be clearly distinguishable from the health profiles of the larger population in which the subpopulation resides. In a 2012 article, I point to "low-risk islands within seas of high risk" unacknowledged in public health programs targeting racial groups as high-risk population lumps: "White" people targeted by genetic testing guidelines for their risk of cystic fibrosis (American College of Obstetricians and Gynecologists Committee on Genetics 2011) and "African Americans" targeted by US government dietary guidelines recommending dietary salt reduction (U.S. Department of Agriculture and U.S. Department of Health and Human Services 2010) due to elevated hypertension rates (Valles 2012: 405). However, each program fails to respond to the data indicating that there are distinct known subpopulations within the racial groups that have radically lower risks: White people of Finnish ancestry have cystic fibrosis rates roughly ten times lower than the White average, and the foreign-born Black population in the US, on average, has far better cardiovascular health than the African American population (and better cardiovascular health than US-born Whites) (Valles 2012). Lumping these known and identifiable low-risk populations into high-risk aggregate population lumps effectively ignores relevant evidence that could be used to more effectively direct resources to the populations that are actually at high risk.

The lumping vs. splitting problem will continue to vex population health practitioners just as it vexes other life scientists trying to make sense of the fuzzy clustering patterns of the biological world. I offer two epistemic/evidentiary heuristics as guidelines to help population health practitioners faced by the question of how fine-grained to make their population partitions. I base the first recommendation on a chapter in the foundational population health science volume, *Why are Some People Healthy and Others Not?* The second guideline is based on advice offered by a philosopher of biology and medicine drawing lessons from the disputed use of racial groupings in biomedicine.

Hertzman, Frank and Evans advocate for an epistemic strategy that takes its goal to be the identification of hidden social determinants buried beneath the surface of a population. As they put it:

> A population can be partitioned according to any number of different characteristics. But the interesting partitions are those which consistently demonstrate clear heterogeneity of health status across their subgroups in many diverse settings.
>
> (Hertzman et al. 1994: 75)

We should try dividing up populations in different ways, looking for discernible and actionable patterns until we encounter some partition scheme that shows a distribution of health outcomes that persist after controlling for confounding variables. They give the example of socioeconomic status's positive correlation with good health. Only by splitting the population into socioeconomic subgroups did Marmot's Whitehall Study make its groundbreaking discovery of the gradient of health. As reviewed in Chapter 2, that gradient manifests across the globe in very different societies with very different cultures, environments, social structures, etc.; the "status syndrome" is a robust cross-cultural health phenomenon (Marmot 2004).

Essentially, Hertzman et al. direct us to design research variables with the goal of uncovering Rose's "causes of incidence," discussed in Chapter 5 (Rose 1992; Hertzman et al. 1994). That is, we should partition populations into whatever lumps best help us to find the causes that lead some populations to have good health, while other populations have poor health—*The Determinants of Health of Populations*, to use the phrasing in the subtitle of the foundational population health science book in which Hertzman's chapter appears (Evans et al. 1994). Between Rose's advice to turn attention to these causes and the aforementioned foundational book's similar prioritizing of it, it is clearly a central priority of population health science to identify the causes of health heterogeneity between populations.

The lumping vs. splitting problem is, for all population life sciences, inherently a problem of grappling with the reality of variation. Population health science takes a unique angle on lumping vs. splitting by making it a disciplinary goal to uncover the *causes* of populations' widely varying health. Adapting this point into a methodological guideline, I offer the following: *During population health research and interventions, when it is unclear whether to lump/aggregate or split/disaggregate a given population in order to choose a specific population grouping as the object of research/intervention, practitioners should choose the population grouping(s) that appears most likely to uncover "causes of incidence" of health and illness.*

I offer the above guideline as the first half of a pair of guidelines; the second deals more directly with the ethical implications of the methodological question of lumping/splitting, drawing from the work of philosopher of medicine Koffi Maglo. Maglo has formulated a rule for the use of race in medicine, but this can be adapted as a general rule of research design to help constrain the overabundance of possible choices facing population health practitioners trying to choose population groupings.

> The Excluded Beneficiary Rule: In the context of theory-choice, the most robust model or clinical trial concept is the one that meets the requirement of improving the status of orphan populations.
>
> (Maglo 2010: 367)

Maglo's concept of the excluded beneficiary rule translates well into a new general population health guideline for solving the problem of deciding which scale of population grouping scheme is the right one, which lumps or splits to use. The adapted guideline is: *During population health research and interventions, when it is unclear whether to lump/aggregate or split/disaggregate a given population, one should choose the population grouping that appears most likely to promote the welfare of population segments whose needs are most underserved.* This may seem like a narrow position on philosophy's equity debates over prioritarianism, health maximization, and related questions of how to balance the needs of the many and the needs of the most disadvantaged (see Chapter 7). But, it is important to remember that this guideline is triggered when practitioners are left in a state of uncertainty about how to proceed otherwise. I am not trying to take a stance on Rawls' famously controversial difference principle, which condones social inequalities if the largest gains are directed to those who are the most disadvantaged (Rawls 1999). Chapter 7 will elaborate on this and related issues.

The high-risk approach vs. the population approach

Keyes and Galea's book *Population Health Science* wastes no time setting up Geoffrey Rose as the field's founder; the book is dedicated to Rose, whose "insights laid the foundation for population health science" (Keyes and Galea 2016). While Chapter 2 gives a more expansive account of the history of population health sciences, I wholeheartedly agree that Rose was, and remains, one of the most crucial contributors to population health theory and that his insights remain acutely relevant more than two decades after his death in 1993. Indeed, Chapter 5 and the immediately preceding section of this chapter both strongly endorse his recommendation to direct attention to "causes of incidence" (Rose 1985, 1992)—the causes of health disparities between populations. Perhaps his most elegantly simple and pivotal contribution to population health theory was articulating the benefits and drawbacks of two very different strategies for promoting public health; the high-risk strategy advocated in Canada's internationally influential proto-population health science document, the Lalonde Report (Lalonde 1974) vs. the under-appreciated population approach that had proven effective in the history of public health (targeting the entire population for a modest shift toward better health, without concentrating resources on the most risky subpopulations) (Rose 1985). This connects with the wider political philosophy debate over egalitarianism (the pursuit of fair and equal health; Daniels 2008), prioritarianism (giving strong precedence to those most in need; Temkin 2003), and the goal of maximizing health (as opposed to the goal of promoting some sufficient threshold level of health; Schramme 2016), as discussed in Chapter 7.

In work culminating in his classic text, *The Strategy of Preventive Medicine*, Rose identified two distinct methods for pursuing health promotion, each with benefits and drawbacks (Rose 1992). The "high-risk approach" targets public health resources at those who have the highest risks; people with family histories of diabetes have their metabolic health tested more often, university students living in crowded residence halls are vaccinated for meningitis, etc. Rose points out that such interventions are economically efficient insofar as they direct resources precisely where needed and are most likely to inspire buy-in from both caregivers and those being cared for (Rose 1985). Unfortunately, that approach eventually transformed into an illustration of the biomedical model's limits. Rose uses the example of mass screening of cholesterol levels as a means of assessing and addressing heart disease risk, casting doubt on its predicative power for individuals and its overall value as a population-level intervention (Rose 1985). A recent meta-analysis of the efficacy of risk-screening tests of asymptomatic people (mammograms, prostate specific antigen, blood sugar, etc.), has found disappointing net benefits:

> Among currently available screening tests for diseases where death is a common outcome, reductions in disease-specific mortality are uncommon and reductions in all-cause mortality are very rare or non-existent.
>
> (Saquib et al. 2015)

As Rose explains, pouring resources into tests and risk estimates is efficient in the short term, but does nothing to address the underlying causes of incidence that make some populations more prone to problems than others (Rose 1985). For example, blood sugar tests can, at best, identify when single patients are beginning to show diabetic symptoms and although they hold promise that early detections will add up to a significant benefit for the population, they do nothing to illuminate or address the linked set of environmental–cultural–behavioral causes that lead some populations to have vastly higher rates of diabetes than others.

On the other hand, the "population strategy" targets the entire population, including the low-risk and the healthy (Rose 1985); automobile fuel efficiency standards improve air quality for all and campaigns to socially de-normalize smoking change the risk and reward context of every individual's decision about whether to smoke. However, these efforts are prone to the "prevention paradox," under which individual population members get such tiny individual benefits that the efforts inspire little motivation among the population members and those tasked with carrying out the interventions (Rose 1985). Rose famously favored the population strategy, given the total risks and benefits.

In his chapter for *Why Are Some People Healthy and Others Not?*, Renaud warned that a population strategy can still leave an inequitable health gradient in place (Renaud 1994). As seen in Chapter 2, it was not until the 1980s and after that Marmot's Whitehall study, and later replications, firmly established the epidemiological phenomenon of the health–socioeconomic status gradient ("the status syndrome") that shapes everyone's health, from the wealthiest segments of the wealthiest societies to the poorest segments of the poorest societies (Marmot et al. 1984; Marmot 2004). Creating new "population strategy" inter-ventions to slightly raise up everyone in an entire population ("particularly with respect to alcohol, tobacco and diet") will not change the fact that some people were already higher up than others (Renaud 1994: 322). Frohlich and Potvin have continued this critique and argued that a population strategy can actually make inequities worse (Frohlich and Potvin 2008). Recalling Chapter 2, one reason is that Rose's "approach is blind to the crucial effect of the life course," including the fact that we cannot manipulate risk exposures atomistically—(Frohlich and Potvin 2008: 219); for example, the health risks I face at age 35 are highly contingent on the health risks I faced in preceding decades. This point is related to Frohlich and Potvin's simultaneous advocacy of fundamental causes, in that they urge consideration of the interconnectedness of risk patterns.

Frohlich and Potvin endorse Link and Phelan's "fundamental cause" notion (Phelan and Link 2005; Link and Phelan 1995). They find value in Rose's recommendation to pursue a population strategy but point out that we should, in parallel, also attend to the needs of "vulnerable populations" because of the distributions of health risks and the benefits of health interventions (Frohlich and Potvin 2008). "Vulnerable populations" (e.g., socially marginalized racial/ethnic minorities) are populations whose members' life courses are subjected to a multiple overlapping of risk factors (e.g., diet, de facto segregation in neighborhoods with poor air quality, inadequate recreation facilities for exercise). Indeed, the importance of recognizing overlapping social harms among those with multiple marginalized identities are a key justification of intersectionality theory, especially given that the causal dynamics might be non-additive in nature (Bright et al. 2016)—that is, the health risks faced by being a Black gay man in a culture dominated by straight White people is not reducible to the additive risks of being a Black man (subjected to inequitable distribution of inherited wealth, etc.) plus the risks of being a gay man (subjected to legal or illegal employment discrimination, etc.). Vulnerable populations, by virtue of their social position, are impacted by many negative social and physical determinants, and addressing these social determinants (e.g., desegregation) is different than ineffectually chasing individual risk factors (Frohlich and Potvin 2008). Frohlich and Potvin point to data accumulated after Rose's death, indicating that when population health strategies are applied they can worsen inequities by concentrating benefits among those who have the most resources; one cited example is smoking education campaigns that make a bigger impact on people with higher education levels) (Frohlich and Potvin 2008).

While population strategy interventions are not a panacea, their faults can be mitigated. McLaren et al. argue that Frohlich and Potvin are too quick to cast aspersions on a population strategy since it is not necessarily the case that every population strategy intervention will worsen health inequities (McLaren et al. 2010). More specifically, interventions that seek to modify *individual behavior* are prone to differential and potentially inequitable uptake, whereas Rose's favorite sorts of inventions—the "radical" ones (Rose 1985)—target the *upstream socioenvironmental contexts* in which individual behaviors occur. These interventions are less prone to the inequitable distribution of benefits; for example, water fluoridation has narrowed the socioeconomic disparities in tooth loss and other oral health measures (McLaren et al. 2010).

Subsequent work by Link and Phelan (whom Frohlich and Potvin had cited) helps to chart a means of narrowing down the application of the population strategy while simultaneously addressing Frohlich and Potvin's urging that we "ensure that vulnerable populations are not left behind in the improvement of population health" (Frohlich and Potvin 2008: 219). Phelan et al. argue that we can avoid the problem of neglecting the most disadvantaged and vulnerable by using population strategies that do not require members of the population to have resources in order to benefit from them (Phelan et al. 2010). They give the example of two potential population strategies: decreasing birth defects by creating education campaigns advising all pregnant women to consume folic acid vs. adding folic acid to grain products during manufacturing (Phelan et al. 2010). While some have expressed concerns that folic acid fortification could push some above the upper safe limit of the vitamin (e.g., those who take additional vitamin supplement pills; Reynolds 2016), there is ample evidence that fortification is a very effective means of reducing birth defects (Atta et al. 2016). Both are broadly cast population strategies and both have the potential to shift the mean health of the population by impacting every birth, but the latter intervention has the crucial additional virtue of helping even those who would get missed by an education campaign, such as people with low access to healthcare education materials.

In the previous section, on lumping vs. splitting, I concluded by arguing that two guidelines should serve as heuristics as we decide how to proceed when facing a conundrum over whether to focus on a large population lump or a smaller population split. Those guidelines can be better understood in combination with the lessons of the Rose debate in this section. To briefly recap, I argued in the previous section that we should prioritize population groupings that: (1) help us to uncover "causes of incidence" (another Rose innovation), and (2) serve the needs of subgroups who would otherwise be most drastically underserved. The first guideline's rationale is based in part on the Rose debate's lessons that (a) there is very wide variation in health risks and (b) interventions that do not radically address underlying causes of health are "palliative and temporary—not radical" (Rose 1985: 36). However, adopting Rose's population strategy can also make inequity worse, which leads us to the second guideline. Phelan et al. argue that we should "prioritize the development of interventions that do not entail the use of resources or that minimize the relevance of resources" in order to avoid leaving behind under-resourced segments of the population as we shift forward the mean health of the population (Phelan et al. 2010: S37). I find it hasty to leap to this level of specificity of advice, and instead share Frohlich and Potvin's more generalized concern for what happens to the most disadvantaged margins of the population. If a proposed population strategy intervention were to require resources *and those resources were adequately provided to all*—especially those most desperately needing those resources—then I would find the intervention to be suitable and equitable.

Based on the above, I offer this guideline: *population health interventions using the population strategy are acceptable and desirable, but only if the interventions are unlikely to underserve subpopulations that currently lack any of the resources needed to benefit from the intervention.* I see my recommendation as very much in line with Phelan et al.'s advice (Phelan et al. 2010) and interpret that advice as a means of achieving the population strategy goal I articulate in the second lumping vs. splitting guideline provided above (*During population health research and interventions, when it is unclear whether to lump/aggregate or split/disaggregate a given population, one should choose the population grouping that appears most likely to promote the welfare of population segments whose needs are most underserved*).

Decentering the healthcare system to promote population health vs. expanding outward from the healthcare system

This chapter is divided into four vexing methodological questions that population health efforts must contend with. The preceding sections laid out two related questions about strategies for population health research and practice, united by the common thread of the need to address population heterogeneity and balance the needs of different segments of a given population. These methodological questions must be answered in light of two overarching challenges that are also methodological, but at the scale of how population health science navigates its relationships with theoretical systems and practices that are partly likeminded but which disagree with population health science about crucial theoretical matters. This section will focus on the particular trade-offs that population health science faces as a radical scientific program that exists in a world where many key institutions, programs, policymakers, and scientists agree that population health promotion efforts need reforming, but are unwilling to be so radical. The danger is that population health science must balance pragmatic accomplishment of desirable goals without reinforcing undesirable elements of older models of health science. This section will illustrate the general problem by examining an illustrative case of this sort of tension.

The "Triple Aim" framework has become influential in health scholarship by placing population health promotion as one of three co-equal goals, all while focusing on the healthcare sector as the locus of population health promotion (Berwick et al. 2008). This, creates a conundrum for population health scientists, who clearly support the goal of population health promotion, but whose theoretical commitments reject the presumption that healthcare is the proper focus of interventions and who have much reason to be suspicious that population health ought to be pursued as a co-equal goal with the Triple Aim's two other objectives—both of which are healthcare system management aims: "improving the individual experience of care" (in healthcare) and "reducing the per capita costs of care for populations" (Berwick et al. 2008: 760).

The Triple Aim is a suite of policy goals developed at the Institute for Healthcare Improvement: "improving the patient experience of care, improving the health of populations, and reducing the per capita cost of health care" (Lewis 2014).[1] It has played an influential role in the developing scholarship of, and applied efforts in, "population health management" (Whittington et al. 2015). The tension between the population health framework and the Triple Aim can be understood in part as a question of how radically population health researchers and practitioners should reject the powerful role of the healthcare system in population health promotion. As shown in Chapter 2, population health science is a field built upon the gradual realization that scholars had previously over-estimated the degree to which health is determined by the healthcare sector's activities, and underestimated the roles played by everyday social lives and their environmental contexts. Hence, there is a tension between the population health framework and any methodology for population health promotion that centers around the healthcare system. As Kindig and Isham put it in a debate over what healthcare can do to serve overall population health: "our succinct, summary response would be '… but it's not primarily about medical care'" (Kindig and Isham 2014: 56).

The Triple Aim raises a thorny methodological challenge. On the one hand, it acknowledges, "improving health is a challenge that requires the engagement of partners across the community to address the broader determinants of health" (Lewis 2014). But on the other, it commits the same unfortunate conflation of health and healthcare that Arah so pointedly warns against (Arah 2009), Chapters 3 and 4 showed how this common conflation has led to errors in how health is defined and approached in practice. The Triple Aim has been offered as a means of "improving the U.S. health care system," by the Institute for *Health-care* Improvement; healthcare remains at the center of the Triple Aim even if it is committed to expanding population health promotion beyond the borders of contemporary healthcare institutions. Berwick et al. offered a widely cited intro-duction to the Triple Aim in 2008 (Berwick et al. 2008), which fittingly garnered qualified praise from David Kindig, one of population health science's foremost communicators, citing the same sort of error decried by Arah.

> while Berwick and his coauthors suggest that the Triple Aim is in part to improve health rather than health care, almost [all] of the paper is really limited to reform of the health care system.

> (Kindig 2008)

This combination of overriding concern with healthcare and the high priority placed on cost control return renew a long-standing philosophical question in population health science discourse: how legitimate is it to foreground economic benefits of population health improvement if population health science is more concerned with the direct humanistic benefits of promoting populations' health? In 2003, Kickbusch, a leading scholar of social determinants of health, pointed out the tensions between the humanistic and economic arguments for the popu-lation health framework (Kickbusch 2003). Poland et al. had pointed out similar tensions in a critique of Evans and Stoddart's keystone population health article, arguing that their focus on the economic inefficiencies of the biomedical model actually gave an argument to conservative policymakers who wish to find ways of chipping away at healthcare social welfare programs (Poland et al. 1998; Evans and Stoddart 1990). Chapter 2 discussed Szreter's historical argument that McKeown's data on the weakness of healthcare as a determinant of health ended up serving similar conservative policy ends (Szreter 2003, 2005: 23–42). By contrast, in 2003 Kickbusch already saw signs that "commitment to values such as equity, participation, solidarity, sustainability, and accountability" were starting to make their way into "the population health debate, which focuses on an economic rather than a humanistic rationale" (Kickbusch 2003: 385).

In 2014, Sharfstein darkly surmised that "'population health,' as a term, appears to be losing its connection with why it was defined a decade ago" (Sharfstein 2014: 642).

> Instead of serving as a light to illuminate the world outside the boundaries of medical treatment, the term "population health" has become a mirror that reflects back to the leaders of the health care system various ideas for initiatives under their control.
>
> (Sharfstein 2014: 642)

Population health promotion efforts done without population health science's firm commitment to addressing the full range of health causes in social life can fall victim to the classic error that when one's only tool is a hammer, all problems begin to look like nails. For many members of the healthcare sector, health problems all look like problems for healthcare to solve.

A philosophical dispute lies beneath the surface of the simultaneous successes of the population health framework in general and of population health pursued under the aegis of the Triple Aim. Michael Stoto (2013) pinpoints the tension as a matter of whether it is population health improvement as Kindig and Stoddart (2003) claimed, or whether it is an "instrumental goal" for those primarily concerned with improving the efficiency of the healthcare system. The Triple Aim has become a powerful force in the US healthcare reform process (Lewis 2014), which forces population health science scholars and practitioners to decide whether they will treat the Triple Aim as a competitor or an ally. I argue that the tractability of the debate over the Triple Aim's relationship with the population health framework depends on two factors.

First, there need to be more voices like Sharfstein's, Kickbusch's, and Stoto's, bringing careful scholarly analyses of the tensions as well as commonalities. Stoto helps to show that the two sides of the dispute—population health promotion as an end in itself vs. population health promotion as an instrumental means of healthcare sector reform—are united by a shared understanding of the nature and causation of health and health causation, in that both sides take "holistic" approaches to health by understanding health as a life course process that must be measured by more than just health outcomes (the distal end points such as mortality rates of specific disease, as discussed in Chapter 4) (Stoto 2013). Moreover, Stoto argues, the two sides share an acknowledgment that upstream causal factors (social determinants, etc.) need to be addressed, and they also share a commitment to reducing inequitable health disparities (Stoto 2013). We must understand what is, and is not, involved in this disagreement.

Second, there is reason to be optimistic if more of the conservative or piecemeal health reform efforts continue to cede ground to the more radical population health science. The Institute for Healthcare Improvement (IHI) says that it has focused on standard healthcare settings, but aspires to expand its framework in a way that makes it appear to closely align with the population health framework.

> IHI will continue to broaden its understanding of the Triple Aim and its meaning beyond the healthcare system: to population and community health, the experience of care and health for the individual, and per capita cost of care paired with a focus on the economic vitality of the community.
>
> (Lewis 2014)

This is a very encouraging aspiration, insofar as it changes tack toward even more radical social justice gains (especially an explicit concern for communities) and further embraces health's connection to the upstream causal factors tied to a community's economic welfare.

Much is at stake in population health science's collective decisions about whether and how it will work alongside potential allies who have partially diverging philosophical commitments. Historically, the fate of the field of Social Medicine serves as a cautionary example. As seen in Chapters 1 and 2, all three are rooted in radical leftist political efforts to promote health equity, including direct leadership roles in these efforts played by two of the leading leftist figures of the nineteenth and twentieth centuries, Friedrich Engels and Salvador Allende. But, the inevitable practical question is which approaches to health promotion remain compatible with forming fruitful collaborations with people and institutions who are not radical leftists. Social Medicine remains overtly leftist in its politics, partly thanks to leadership by Emily and Sidney Kark, and Paul Farmer—as is fittingly articulated (in a socialist magazine) by the managers of the Social Medicine Portal website and its associated open-access peer-reviewed journal, *Social Medicine* (Anderson et al. 2005).

The staunch anti-corporate messaging of Social Medicine effectively precludes intersectoral collaboration with the for-profit sector, which thus shuts down productive relationships with the wealthy and powerful biomedical industry (pharmaceutical companies, healthcare insurers in regions where private insurance is available, etc.). Taking an even more uncompromising position, The People's Health Movement is openly hostile to the very presence of the private sector in healthcare, similarly serving to limit its ability to work with one of the key sectors that can contribute to population health promotion (Schuftan 2017). Meanwhile, it is rather dogmatic in its relationship to the government sector—its opposition to the "USA-led" War on Terror appears to be more an extension of the political leftism of the group than its specific health goals (even though the War on Terror has health repercussions). That stance puts the entire movement into immediate tension with the US and many other militarily allied nations that together control a huge proportion of the resources (monetary, intellectual, etc.) that must be redirected for effective and equitable population health promotion (Schuftan 2017).

Evidence-based medicine vs. public health pragmatism

Population health science's tension with evidence-based medicine is related to its tension with efforts that center general population health promotion efforts on the healthcare sector. Evidence-based medicine (EBM) does not so explicitly commit to the conceptual error of conflating health and healthcare the way that the Triple Aim has (Kindig 2008). EBM has raised a key methodological problem for population health science by setting influential new standards for what qualifies as good evidence of whether and how an intervention is efficacious. Now, the nascent population health science needs to determine whether, and how much, it will cast its lot with EBM's contentions about what good health science looks like.

Evidence-based medicine is a self-styled "new paradigm" working to effect a (Kuhnian scientific) revolution in what qualifies as good medical evidence, how medical evidence is collected, and how medical evidence directs clinical decision-making (Evidence-Based Medicine Working Group 1992; Solomon 2015). Philosopher Jeremy Howick explains that EBM has had multiple meanings from its earliest days, but all versions give far higher weight to evidence collected systematically in comparative effectiveness trials, preferably randomized controlled trials, as well as systematic evidence syntheses of such evidence (e.g., a meta-analysis of several randomized controlled trials that each compare the health outcomes of patients taking Drug A vs. those taking Drug B for the treatment of Disease C) (Howick 2011). This evidence is prioritized over less strictly collected forms of evidence, such as an individual/group's accumulated clinical wisdom or its professional prestige, or the use of mechanistic reasoning (e.g., inferring that Drug A is superior to Drug B because Drug A's molecules accumulate more selectively in the tissues affected by Disease C, and hence ought to reduce side effects in off-target tissues) (Howick 2011). Evidence-based medicine is a hot topic in the philosophy of medicine, and philosophers have leveled a plethora of critiques against features such as hierarchical understandings of evidence (Borgerson 2009), its overconfidence in meta-analyses (Stegenga 2011), and inadequate attention to the social dynamics of dissent, consensus, and decision-making (Solomon 2015). It is beyond the scope of this book to take stances on each of these and other critiques.

Continuing the last section's discussion of Berwick (a leader of the Triple Aim effort), an examination of his stance on EBM sheds light on the ambiguous relationship of population health science and the evidence-based medicine paradigm. Solomon's philosophical analysis of EBM points to Berwick as a key figure, both in developing EBM and in later articulating its limitations (Solomon 2015: 2–3). Berwick had:

lamented that we have "overshot the mark" and created "intellectual hegemony" with evidence-based medicine (Berwick 2005) … His fear is that
evidence-based medicine will lead only to conservative innovation and be
limited to interventions ready to go into clinical trials.

(Solomon 2015: 2–3)

This conservatism is problematically limiting, even for innovations pursued
within traditional healthcare contexts, as Berwick says. It is all the more limiting
for the population health framework and its emphasis on upstream determinants
of health, the social/environmental causes that manifest in a myriad of health
outcomes that vary by context. For example, racism is a cause with devastating
health effects, but it manifests via many intermediary mechanisms ranging from
physician implicit biases leading to over-treatment, under-treatment and other
clinical errors (Chapman et al. 2013; Paradies et al. 2015) to exposing minority
communities to waterborne contaminants because of racist political disenfran-
chisement and neglect of community infrastructure (e.g., the infamous Flint
Water Crisis afflicting my Michigan neighbors) (Krieger 2016; Sherwin 2017;
Michigan Civil Rights Commission 2017).

As Solomon indicates in the passage above, Berwick's "pragmatic" concern
about EBM's limitations is key. Marmot's UN Commission on the Social
Determinants of Health illustrates both why the population health framework is
theoretically aligned with evidence-based medicine and also why EBM's preferred sources of data—randomized controlled trials and meta-analyses
thereof—are only sometimes able to provide the evidence that population health
framework activities require. The Commission points out that, "interventions
such as the development and implementation of laws that protect gender equity,
for instance, cannot be randomized across countries" (Commission on Social
Determinants of Health 2008: 42). As a result, there is a dearth of randomized
controlled experimental data on interventions that target social determinants
and other upstream social causes of health, and those that do exist are prone to
falling short of EBM standards. For example, a 2015 systematic review and
meta-analysis of "Unconditional cash transfers for assistance in humanitarian
disasters: effect on use of health services and health outcomes in low- and
middle-income countries" found three studies that met its review criteria but all
three studies were rated as having very low quality as evidence. The Commission and other population health science efforts have learned to carry on without
such data.

Had the Commission made a decision to rely on evidence solely from well-
controlled experiments, this would be a short report with only biomedical
evidence-based recommendations and the conclusion that more research
is needed. Equity and social justice, even health, would not have
progressed much.

(Commission on Social Determinants of Health 2008: 42)

Nevertheless, it is intriguing to see that the Commission expresses a preference for EBM's favored type of evidence (randomized controlled trials), even though such evidence is usually unavailable. Inaction is not an ethically acceptable option, so the Commission uses the best evidence at its disposal. This point is echoed elsewhere, such as Lie and Miller's advocacy of using observational data alongside randomized controlled trials when deciding whether to recommend male circumcision as a means of reducing risk of HIV transmission (Lie and Miller 2011). There is currently an effort to work toward correcting that evidence lacuna, though that effort's ongoing challenges show why reconciling the epistemic/evidentiary tension between population health science and EBM will be even more difficult than it first appears.

The influential Robert Wood Johnson Foundation has recently made a push for evidence-based population health research, under its funding program, "Evidence for Action: Investigator-Initiated Research to Build a Culture of Health." A social scientific study of the disputes that arose during the creation of the program to develop "evidence-based population health" illuminates the unresolved philosophical questions of method that make it difficult to create an EBM-type evidence base for population health science interventions (Gottlieb et al. 2016). One finding of the analysis is that the (de)centralization of population health science efforts will have an enormous impact on its future. EBM's record of successes and influence has been driven in large part by support from regulators and funders such as the Centers for Medicare & Medicaid Services in the US (Berwick 2016) and The National Institute for Health and Care Excellence in the UK (Solomon 2015). These sorts of agencies are able to strongly constrain medical practice through regulatory and funding powers. By contrast, population health science is built upon a rejection of the notion that we can rely primarily on the healthcare system as a means of achieving health gains in the population. Even governments will have limited control over many of the diffuse population health promotion efforts, such as population health nutrition initiatives spearheaded by charitable organizations. As Chapter 4 argued, population health science is, and should be, philosophically committed to studying and intervening upon health no matter where its determinants lay—often healthcare and government will have minimal roles. As Chapter 8 will further argue, this state of affairs makes it all the more essential that population health science strives for non-hierarchical collaborative relationships between the various sectors (e.g., governments and non-profits) and experts, for example, epidemiologists with statistical expertise and non-scientist population members with expertise in their own communities' social dynamics (McHugh 2015). The consequence is that there are limited means by which EBM standards can be externally imposed on population health scientists. In other words, EBM has become embedded in healthcare thanks to institutional factors that have less sway over population health science.

Even if there were a new influx of EBM research on social determinants of health and other population health science priorities, then researchers would just be led back to the population heterogeneity problems discussed in the first half of the chapter (in addition to the Triple Aim problem). Solomon shows in detail why even rigorously collected EBM-type clinical data still leaves us with difficult epistemic and ethical decisions to make due to human variation (Solomon 2015: 143–148). A clear signal that Drug A has a higher mean efficacy and fewer mean serious side effects than Drug B, does not mean that all subpopulations will respond similarly. A classic case is the evidence that certain antidepressants seem to increase risk of suicide in the subgroup of children and adolescents, but not in older patients (McGoey 2009). In other words, even if the population health framework had access to a wealth of the randomized controlled trial data valued so highly by EBM, this would still leave the population health science struggling with the other issues in this chapter.

Conclusion

This chapter has divided up the challenges facing the population health framework into four philosophical disputes over methodology. The first two disputes, lumping vs. splitting and the high-risk strategy vs. the population strategy, turn out to be closely related. In the former, I recommend that in cases of uncertainty about how to divide up a given population, we should take it as a heuristic to try to satisfy two criteria: (1) use population divisions that are likely to uncover Rose's so-called "causes of incidence" that shape population-level health patterns, and (2) use population divisions that are likely to serve the needs of those whose needs are most underserved. The latter criterion is partly justified by the weaknesses that have attended Rose's two competing strategies (Rose 1992).

The next two ongoing conundrums for the population health framework involve reaching a decision about how to interact with two other movements that emerged out of frustrations with the status quo of biomedicine: the Triple Aim and evidence-based medicine. The Triple Aim and EBM frameworks have developed such that they diverge from, and converge with, the population health framework in curious ways. The Triple Aim is by definition committed to population health improvement, but it pursues this as a means of trying to rescue a healthcare system that is centered on the biomedical model—a commitment very much in tension with the population health framework's historical trajectory as a rejection of the idea that the healthcare system can lay at the center of effective population health efforts. Yet, the Triple Aim leaders have also shown an openness to broadening the Triple Aim so that even if the healthcare system remains at its center, the healthcare system may occupy less of the total territory after the borders of Triple Aim's domain of interest are pushed outward. As a result, I contend that the population health framework and the Triple Aim can be valuable allies in their common goals. Theoretically, EBM should have no deep-seated dispute with the population health framework, and this has yielded the favorable EBM views of some population health scholars noted above. After all, it is a movement that insists we pay far more attention to population-level health data (i.e. epidemiological evidence). In practice, though, the EBM movement has generated very sparse population health-relevant data that would qualify as high-quality data under EBM standards. Population health science has learned to live without the benefit of randomized controlled trial data. Population health science is right to be so pragmatic, and I offer this chapter as guidance for how to balance that pragmatism with the methodological decisions faced in population health science practice. To illustrate the themes in this chapter, the following case study will examine the heterogeneous and perplexing health of global migrants.

Case study: the heterogeneous health of migrants

Research on the population health of migrants has developed considerably in recent years. Migration itself is nothing new, even mass migration—recall that the case studies in Chapter 2 and Chapter 3 each deal with the interactions between the descendants of (colonial) migrants and the indigenous populations that preceded them. The rate of international migration (let alone migration within countries) is growing faster than the total human population (United Nations 2016). Due to advances in transportation technologies, rates of migration will likely continue (Florey et al. 2007). Figure 6.1 depicts the 2017 Day without an Immigrant protest in Washington DC, opposing the growth of anti-immigrant sentiments in the US. Even within countries there can be massive migration shifts, such as the global trend toward urbanization (the flow of migrants from rural environments to urban ones) (Florey et al. 2007).

Yet, migrant health is so heterogeneous and so difficult to track via standard administrative data (vital statistics etc. tend to be managed at the national level)

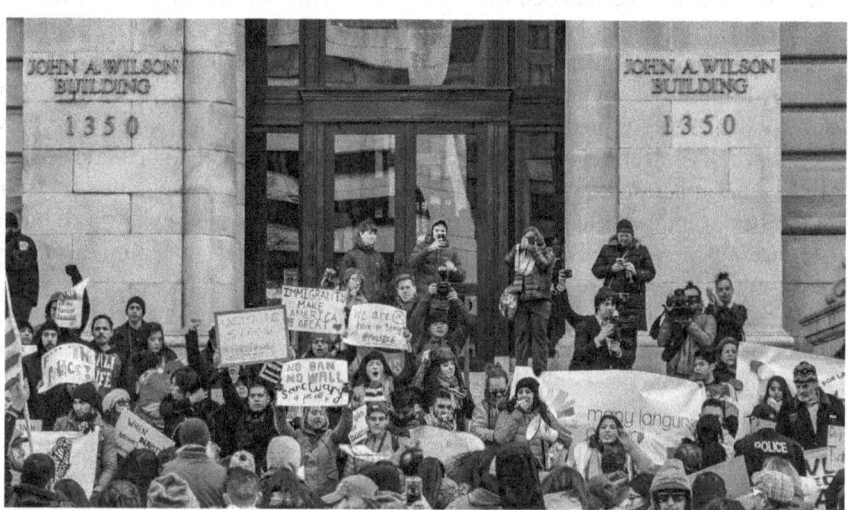

Figure 6.1 "2017.02.16 A Day Without Immigrants, Washington, DC USA 00886" by Ted Eytan. Protestors in front of a government building during the Day Without Immigrants protest and boycott opposing immigration restrictions.

Source: Creative Commons Attribution-ShareAlike 2.0 Generic License. www.flickr.com/photos/taedc/32789288522/in/album-72157678834210020/.

that migrants' health remains a challenge to understand. Adding further intrigue, the Hispanic Paradox phenomenon cited above—the observation that average US Hispanics' health is unexpectedly good, given their low average socio-economic status—is connected in, as yet opaque, ways to a global phenomenon termed the "healthy migrant effect" (Valles 2016). That is, "most migrants, even poor ones, tend to be healthier than the host population" for reasons that remain unclear, though over time migrants' health tends to more and more resemble that of their new neighbors (Bhopal 2014: 96, 143).

Lumping vs. splitting: In an effort to shed light on what makes a large subset of diverse global migrants' health a defensible "lump" for scientific attention, Razum and Twardella offer a conceptual framework for understanding the life course health of migrants who travel from less wealthy regions to wealthier ones: they are somewhat akin to time travelers (Razum and Twardella 2002). In other words, they radically shift their life course trajectories by suddenly altering their behavioral, social, and environmental contexts. When migrating from a low/middle-income country to a high-income country, the shift more particularly takes the form of entering an economically developed context after leaving another context that in many ways resembles the experiences of the ancestors of current populations in economically developed regions. This subset of migrants experiences a rapid and discontinuous shift of life course trajectory even if they retain most of their previous dietary practices and home life dynamics: the food and drink will have different complements of benign and pathogenic microbes, their homes will be situated in totally different communities of non-migrants, their workplaces will have different sets of hazards, etc. Of course, this does not imply that there is only one demographic fate for all populations—such generalizations have rightly inspired critiques of simplistic uses of the concepts "demographic transition" and "epidemiologic transition," as models of the respective shifts in population structure (e.g., declining birth rates in economically developed countries) and of disease burden (e.g., economically developed countries tend to have higher disease burden from chronic cardiovascular and metabolic diseases, rather than infectious diseases) (Weisz and Olszynko-Gryn 2010).

The lumping and splitting decisions made when contending with that massive set of heterogeneous experiences of global migrants, reminds us that we need to be very careful in how we specify our explanatory goals and our choice of phenomenon for a given explanatory task (Valles 2016). While I have previously advised doing more splitting of populations in order to examine the unique experiences of subpopulations, here I urge researchers to first learn the extent of the healthy migrant effect by lumping together all migrants. If there is a common phenomenon that unites together migrants then that must be understood, since it points to the existence of some powerful upstream social force(s) that serve as causes of health incidence, in the Rose sense (Rose 1992). For example, it seems quite possible that migrants across the globe are biased samples of their former populations—the migrants in new locales are relatively healthy because the new locale only sees the healthiest members, the ones who could make the journey (Rubalcava et al. 2008). If this is so then it directs us to examine: the subpopulation of *asylum seekers and other forced migrants*. This subset of migrants indeed seems to have relatively poor health (Bhopal 2014: 9). Dividing up the total population of migrants according to whether they were forced or voluntary serves to direct our attention to how certain variables affect migrant health, especially the health of the most underserved. For example, how does stigma against asylum seekers affect their health, as opposed to surrounding populations that are not subjected to this stigma? Much follow-up research will require more splitting, to search for local sub-phenomena of which health patterns appear in which migrant populations, but it is still vital to first attend to the lump. This fulfills the recommendation proposed above: *During population health research and interventions, when it is unclear whether to lump/aggregate or split/ disaggregate a given population in order to choose a specific population grouping as the object of research/intervention, practitioners should choose the population grouping(s) that appears most likely to uncover "causes of incidence" of health and illness.*

The high-risk approach vs. the population approach: The choice between a high-risk approach vs. a population approach (Rose 1992) is closely related to the problem of lumping vs. splitting since both are matters of whether to tailor research/interventions to the needs of migrant subpopulations or to migrants more generally. Global migration dynamics are famous for their rapid and often unexpected shifts. Accordingly the WHO Regional Director for Europe, Zsuzsanna Jakab, with the backing of the European Public Health Association, favors a population approach. She points out that while we may be tempted to create ad hoc risk management policies in reaction to sudden new threats from Ebola and other diseases, such risk management approaches are unwise. Instead, it would be better to require equitable de jure policies and de facto cultures, making both laws and social norms "hospitable" to all travelers.

> We should focus on ensuring that each and every person on the move has full access to a hospitable environment and, when needed, to high-quality health care, without discrimination on the basis of gender, age, religion, nationality, or race.
>
> (Jakab 2015)

The population health challenges of travel and migration are best addressed by population-wide shifts in the *de jure* health governance systems and de facto attitudes toward foreigners. Nationalism and xenophobia have negative effects for all migrants and travelers, not just the ever-shifting subpopulations who happen to be most vulnerable to abuse in a certain context at a certain moment in time. In the near term there is a rather obvious ethical imperative to care for the needs of refugees and other migrants at especially high risk of harm. But, the unpredictable fluctuations of migration patterns make ad hoc high-risk approach solutions, addressed to specific populations, inferior to a population approach via structural reforms (e.g., lowering the legal barriers at national borders) and cultural reforms (e.g., recognizing travel and migration as components of a free and ethical world).

Each time a migrant crisis emerges (such as the Syrian refugee crisis of the 2010s), the global community struggles to generate an adequate response. Local political and ecological crises are partly inevitable, yet high-risk strategy solutions are forced to react to each crisis as it arises. Even the existence of the recurring problem of migrant crises is predicated on the persistent global failure to build resilient travel and migration governance systems. In sum, targeting the lump population of all migrants through the improvement of overall migration and travel policies would best serve the needs of high-risk migrants, and low-risk migrants besides. Hence, the recommendation I make above is: *During population health research and interventions, when it is unclear whether to lump/aggregate or split/disaggregate a given population, one should choose the population grouping that appears most likely to promote the welfare of population segments whose needs are most underserved.*

Decentering the healthcare system to promote population health vs. expanding out from the healthcare system to promote population health: Migrants are a prime example of a type of population that is inadequately served by most healthcare systems. Migration inevitably creates linguistic or cultural gaps between the population and their (new) neighbors. Obviously, diverse migrant populations have an enormous amount of variation in their particular health statuses and needs. As traced in Chapter 2, the Black Report in the UK and the Lalonde Report learned that universal healthcare is a not a panacea for the health needs of the socioeconomically marginalized populations of a wealthy nation (Black et al. 1980; Lalonde 1974). Wave upon wave of subsequent data has made it abundantly clear that good healthcare is necessary but not sufficient for health.

Migrants have some pressing needs that require healthcare interventions, such as the need for routine tuberculosis screening for migrants coming from regions with high rates of the disease (Loue and Galea 2007, though, even these healthcare needs can only be assessed and addressed if there are equitable and trusting relationships between healthcare providers and migrant populations. Even aside from the need to offer culturally and linguistically appropriate care, migrants cannot be adequately cared for if they are forced "underground" by fear of oppression by the government or their non-migrant neighbors. Empirical data shows that some migrants have in fact delayed TB care in order to avoid unwanted attention from immigration enforcement officials (Loue and Galea 2007). Migrants and their children also face long-term health problems associated with acculturating to wealthier societies and the societies' associated cardiovascular disease (wealthy Western dietary practices, etc.) (Steffen et al. 2006). Migrants are in special need of healthcare soon after migration (for treatment of any conditions acquired in their previous social contexts), but they are in special need of non-healthcare interventions to address the social and environmental determinants affecting their daily lives in the long term. Adoption of metabolically unhealthy "Western" diets, overcrowded housing, high rates of workplace injuries due to economic exploitation, etc. are all matters that need to be addressed primarily outside the healthcare sector. In other words, the long-term health and welfare of migrants depends on health promotion outside the healthcare system and even the healthcare interventions are highly contingent on the removal of legal and social barriers outside the healthcare system.

Evidence-based medicine vs. public health pragmatism: Those who work in migrant health are accustomed to the need to work with relatively sparse and unreliable data, no matter how hard they try to acquire better data. Data collection strategies on ethnic minorities and migrants is vastly inconsistent even among wealthy nations (e.g., whether and how ethnicity is recorded) (Simon 2012). Bhopal frames the issue in a manner that seems representative of his colleagues who study the population health of migrants. He endorses randomized controlled trials (the preferred evidence-based medicine data) as the best sort of evidence, echoing the Committee on the Social Determinants of Health (Commission on Social Determinants of Health 2008: 42; Bhopal 2014: 217). But, he cautions that it would take decades and billions of pounds in funding to assemble a database on effective interventions for various minority population, including migrant populations, and such an endeavor would of course require the political will to make it happen. The key is that in the meantime we must not succumb to "paralysis" (Bhopal 2014: 217). We can continue to be guided by heuristics such as the knowledge that "human populations are more alike than different," meaning that a pill that works well in non-migrant populations will probably work in migrant populations (Bhopal 2014: 218). By contrast, he says, a more complex intervention such as behavioral guidance given by physicians is unlikely to translate well when applied to a migrant population—sociocultural variations between populations are likely to make the intervention fare quite differently (Bhopal 2014: 218). The status quo is, in fact, so dire that aspirations of an evidence-based database of EBM-type data seem like a pipedream at the moment; we need to first address the grave inequity that migrants are often systematically *excluded* from research, through seemingly benign policies such as requiring that study participants speak English (Bhopal 2014: 218). Perhaps EBM-style data will succeed in becoming increasingly capable of guiding migrant health promotion; in the meantime, population health scientists would be wise to continue being more pragmatic than doctrinaire about what constitutes sufficient evidence.

Notes

1 Harking back to Chapter 1's discussion of "population health" as a science, model, a research program, a paradigm, a framework, etc.—the Institute of Health improvement explicitly asks that the Triple Aim also be referred to as a framework rather than a model or a concept, though this preference is not explained (Lewis 2014).

Works cited

American College of Obstetricians and Gynecologists Committee on Genetics. (2011) Update on carrier screening for cystic fibrosis. *Obstetrics and Gynecology* 117, 1028–1031.

Anderson, M. R., Smith, L. and Sidel, V. W. (2005) What is social medicine? *Monthly Review*, 56. Available at: https://monthlyreview.org/2005/01/01/what-is-social-medicine/.

Arah, O. A. (2009) On the relationship between individual and population health. *Medicine, Health Care and Philosophy* 12, 235–244.

Atta, C. A. M., Fiest, K. M., Frolkis, A. D., et al. (2016) Global birth prevalence of spina bifida by folic acid fortification status: A systematic review and meta-analysis. *American Journal of Public Health* 106, e24-e34.

Berwick, D. M. (2005) Broadening the view of evidence-based medicine. *BMJ Quality & Safety* 14, 315–316.

Berwick, D. M. (2016) Era 3 for medicine and health care. *Journal of the American Medical Association* 315, 1329–1330.

Berwick, D. M., Nolan, T. W. and Whittington, J. (2008) The Triple Aim: Care, health, and cost. *Health Affairs* 27, 759–769.

Bhopal, R. S. (2014) *Migration, Ethnicity, Race, and Health in Multicultural Societies.* Oxford: Oxford University Press.

Black, D., Morris, J., Smith, C. and Townsend, P. (1980) Inequalities in Health: Report of a Research Working Group on Inequalities in Health. London: Department of Health and Social Security.

Borgerson, K. (2009) Why reading the title isn't good enough: An evaluation of the 4S approach to evidence-based medicine. *International Journal of Feminist Approaches to Bioethics* 2, 152–175.

Bright, L. K., Malinsky, D. and Thompson, M. (2016) Causally interpreting intersectionality theory. *Philosophy of Science* 83, 60–81.

Chapman, E. N., Kaatz, A. and Carnes, M. (2013) Physicians and implicit bias: How doctors may unwittingly perpetuate health care disparities. *Journal of General Internal Medicine* 28, 1504–1510.

Commission on Social Determinants of Health. (2008) Closing the Gap in a Generation: Health Equity Through Action on the Social Determinants of Health. Geneva: World Health Organization.

Cortes-Bergoderi, M., Goel, K., Murad, M. H., et al. (2013) Cardiovascular mortality in Hispanics compared to non-Hispanic whites: A systematic review and meta-analysis of the Hispanic paradox. *European Journal of Internal Medicine* 24, 791–799.

Daniels, N. (2008) *Just Health: Meeting Health Needs Fairly.* New York: Cambridge University Press.

Endersby, J. (2009) Lumpers and splitters: Darwin, Hooker, and the search for order. *Science* 326, 1496–1499.

Evans, R. G. and Stoddart, G. L. (1990) Producing health, consuming health care. *Social Science and Medicine* 31, 1347–1363.

Evans, R. G., Barer, M. L. and Marmor, T. R. (1994) *Why Are Some People Healthy and Others Not? The Determinants of Health of Populations.* New York: Aldine De Gruyter.

Evidence-Based Medicine Working Group. (1992) Evidence-based medicine: A new approach to teaching the practice of medicine. *Journal of the American Medical Association* 268, 2420–2425.

Florey, L. S., Galea, S. and Wilson, M. L. (2007) Macrosocial Determinants of Population Health in the Context of Globalization. In: Galea, S. (ed.) *Macrosocial Determinants of Population Health.* New York: Springer Science+Business Media, 15–52.

Frohlich, K. L. and Potvin, L. (2008) Transcending the known in public health practice— the inequality paradox: The population approach and vulnerable populations. *American Journal of Public Health* 98, 216–221.

Gottlieb, L., Glymour, M. M., Kersten, E., et al. (2016) Challenges to an integrated population health research agenda: Targets, scale, tradeoffs and timing. *Social Science & Medicine* 150, 279–285.

Hertzman, C., Frank, J. and Evans, R. G. (1994) Heterogeneities in Health Status and the Determinants of Population Health. In: Evans, R. G., Barer, M. L. and Marmor, T. R. (eds) *Why Are Some People Healthy and Others Not?* New York: Aldine De Gruyter.

Howick, J. H. (2011) *The Philosophy of Evidence-Based Medicine.* Oxford: John Wiley & Sons.

Jakab, Z. (2015) Population movement is a challenge for refugees and migrants as well as for the receiving population. Press release: Copenhagen: WHO Regional Office for Europe. www.euro.who.int/en/health-topics/health-determinants/migration-and-health/news/news/2015/09/population-movement-is-a-challenge-for-refugees-and-migrants-as-well-as-for-the-receiving-population.

Keyes, K. M. and Galea, S. (2016) *Population Health Science.* New York: Oxford University Press.

Kickbusch, I. (2003) The contribution of the World Health Organization to a new public health and health promotion. *American Journal of Public Health* 93, 383–388.

Kindig, D. (2008) Beyond the Triple Aim: Integrating the nonmedical sectors. *Health Affairs Blog.* http://healthaffairs.org/blog/2008/05/19/beyond-the-triple-aim-integrating-the-nonmedical-sectors/.

Kindig, D. and Stoddart, G. (2003) What is population health? *American Journal of Public Health* 93, 380–383.

Kindig, D. A. and Isham, G. (2014) Response from feature authors. *Frontiers of Health Services Management* 30, 56–57.

Krieger, N. (2016) Living and dying at the crossroads: Racism, embodiment, and why theory is essential for a public health of consequence. *American Journal of Public Health* 106, 832–833.

Lalonde, M. (1974) *A New Perspective on the Health of Canadians.* Ottawa, Canada: Health and Welfare Canada.

Lewis, N. (2014) *A Primer on Defining the Triple Aim.* Cambridge, MA: Institute for Healthcare Improvement.

Lie, R. K. and Miller, F. G. (2011) What counts as reliable evidence for public health policy: The case of circumcision for preventing HIV infection. *BMC Medical Research Methodology* 11, 34.

Link, B. G. and Phelan, J. (1995) Social conditions as fundamental causes of disease. *Journal of Health and Social Behavior* 35, 80–94.

Loue, S. and Galea, S. (2007) Migration. In: Galea, S. (ed.) *Macrosocial Determinants of Population Health.* New York: Springer Science+Business Media.

Love, A. C. (2007) The hedgehog, the fox, and reductionism in biology. *Evolution* 61, 2736–2738.

Maglo, K. N. (2010) Genomics and the conundrum of race: Some epistemic and ethical considerations. *Perspectives in Biology and Medicine* 53, 357–372.

Marmot, M. (2004) *The Status Syndrome: How Social Standing Affects Our Health and Longevity*. New York: Henry Holt and Company.

Marmot, M. G., Shipley, M. J. and Rose, G. (1984) Inequalities in death—specific explanations of a general pattern? *The Lancet* 323, 1003–1006.

McGoey, L. (2009) Sequestered evidence and the distortion of clinical practice guidelines. *Perspectives in Biology and Medicine* 52, 203–217.

McHugh, N. A. (2015) *The Limits of Knowledge: Generating Pragmatist Feminist Cases for Situated Knowing*. Albany, NY: SUNY Press.

McLaren, L., McIntyre, L. and Kirkpatrick, S. (2010) Rose's population strategy of prevention need not increase social inequalities in health. *International Journal of Epidemiology* 39, 372–377.

Michigan Civil Rights Commission. (2017) The Flint Water Crisis: Systemic Racism Through the Lens of Flint. Michigan Civil Rights Commission.

Paradies, Y., Ben, J., Denson, N., et al. (2015) Racism as a determinant of health: A systematic review and meta-analysis. *PloS One* 10, e0138511.

Phelan, J. C. and Link, B. G. (2005) Controlling disease and creating disparities: A fundamental cause perspective. *The Journals of Gerontology Series B: Psychological Sciences and Social Sciences* 60, S27–S33.

Phelan, J. C., Link, B. G. and Tehranifar, P. (2010) Social conditions as fundamental causes of health inequalities: Theory, evidence, and policy implications. *Journal of Health and Social Behavior* 51, S28–S40.

Poland, B., Coburn, D., Robertson, A. and Eakin, J. (1998) Wealth, equity and health care: A critique of a "population health" perspective on the determinants of health. *Social Science & Medicine* 46, 785–798.

Rawls, J. (1999) *A Theory of Justice*. Cambridge: Belknap Press.

Razum, O. and Twardella, D. (2002) Time travel with Oliver Twist: Towards an explanation for a paradoxically low mortality among recent immigrants. *Tropical Medicine & International Health* 7, 4–10.

Renaud, M. (1994) The Future: Hygeia vs. Panakeia. In: Evans, R. G., Barer, M. L. and Marmor, T. R. (eds) *Why Are Some People Healthy and Others Not?* New York: Aldine De Gruyter.

Reynolds, E. H. (2016) What is the safe upper intake level of folic acid for the nervous system? Implications for folic acid fortification policies. *European Journal of Clinical Nutrition* 70, 537–540.

Rose, G. (1985) Sick individuals and sick populations. *International Journal of Epidemiology* 14, 32–38.

Rose, G. (1992) *The Strategy of Preventive Medicine*. New York: Oxford University Press.

Rubalcava, L. N., Teruel, G. M., Thomas, D. and Goldman, N. (2008) The healthy migrant effect: New findings from the Mexican Family Life Survey. *American Journal of Public Health* 98, 78–84.

Ruiz, J. M., Steffen, P. and Smith, T. B. (2013) Hispanic mortality paradox: A systematic review and meta-analysis of the longitudinal literature. *American Journal of Public Health* 103, e52–e60.

Saquib, N., Saquib, J. and Ioannidis, J. P. A. (2015) Does screening for disease save lives in asymptomatic adults? Systematic review of meta-analyses and randomized trials. *International Journal of Epidemiology* 44, 264–277.

Schramme, T. (2016) The metric and the threshold problem for theories of health justice: A comment on Venkatapuram. *Bioethics* 30, 19–24.

Schuftan, C. (2017) Peoples Health Movement. In: Quah, S. R. and Cockerham, W. C. (eds) *International Encyclopedia of Public Health.* Second ed. Oxford: Academic Press, 438–441.

Sharfstein, J. M. (2014) The strange journey of population health. *The Milbank Quarterly* 92, 640–643.

Sherwin, B. D. (2017) Pride and prejudice and administrative zombies: How economic woes, outdated environmental regulations, and state exceptionalism failed Flint, Michigan. *University of Colorado Law Review* 88, 653–720.

Simon, P. (2012) Collecting ethnic statistics in Europe: A review. *Ethnic and Racial Studies* 35, 1366–1391.

Solomon, M. (2015) *Making Medical Knowledge.* New York: Oxford University Press.

Steffen, P. R., Smith, T. B., Larson, M. and Butler, L. (2006) Acculturation to Western society as a risk factor for high blood pressure: A meta-analytic review. *Psychosomatic Medicine* 68, 386–397.

Stegenga, J. (2011) Is meta-analysis the platinum standard of evidence? *Studies in History and Philosophy of Biological and Biomedical Sciences* 42, 497–507.

Stoto, M. A. (2013) *Population Health in the Affordable Care Act Era.* Washington, DC: AcademyHealth.

Szreter, S. (2003) The population health approach in historical perspective. *American Journal of Public Health* 93, 421–431.

Szreter, S. (2005) *Health and Wealth.* Rochester, NY: University of Rochester Press.

Temkin, L. S. (2003) Egalitarianism defended. *Ethics* 113, 764–782.

U.S. Department of Agriculture and U.S. Department of Health and Human Services. (2010) Dietary Guidelines for Americans, 2010. In: U.S. Department of Agriculture and U.S. Department of Health and Human Services (eds) 7th Edition ed. Washington, DC: U.S. Government Printing Office.

United Nations. (2016) New York Declaration for Refugees and Migrants. Geneva: United Nations.

Valles, S. A. (2012) Heterogeneity of risk within racial groups, a challenge for public health programs. *Preventive Medicine* 55, 405–408.

Valles, S. A. (2016) The challenges of choosing and explaining a phenomenon in epidemiological research on the "Hispanic Paradox." *Theoretical Medicine and Bioethics* 37, 129–148.

Venkatapuram, S. (2011) *Health Justice: An Argument from the Capabilities Approach.* Malden, MA: Polity Press.

Weisz, G. and Olszynko-Gryn, J. (2010) The theory of epidemiologic transition: The origins of a citation classic. *Journal of the History of Medicine and Allied Sciences* 65, 287–326.

Whittington, J. W., Nolan, K., Lewis, N. and Torres, T. (2015) Pursuing the Triple Aim: The first 7 years. *The Milbank Quarterly* 93, 263–300.

7 Ethics and evidence in the population health equity debates

Introduction: population health science and health equity

Philosophy is gradually recovering from the entrenched disciplinary split between biomedical ethics and the (epistemology/evidence-focused) philosophy of life sciences (Ankeny 2003). As a contribution to a series on the history and philosophy of biology, rather than bioethics or public health ethics, this book is not meant to offer a competitor theory in the vein of Powers and Faden (2006), Daniels (2008), Ruger (2010), Nussbaum (2011), or Venkatapuram (2011). My intended contribution is connected but distinct. Coming from my background as a philosopher of science who also works in bioethics and public health ethics, I wish to clarify the relationship between the theory/practice of population health sciences and the ethical goals of health equity. Taking a step back from the contentious debates over competing health equity theories, this chapter challenges implicit and explicit assumptions that have been directing these debates.

First, I argue that the ethical values of population health science are completely intertwined in evidentiary aspects of the science. Next, I argue that the disputes over the precise meaning and moral foundations of health equity neither will, nor should, end with one ethical framework "winning"; I then argue that this ethical pluralism does not doom efforts to actually work toward health equity in the world. Rather than disputing the meaning of health equity, I argue that equitable health practice is better served by setting in place inclusive participatory processes for making health equity decisions. These processes, not top-down imposition of scholars' predetermined equity definitions, are the proper drivers of equitable health promotion and health governance. Indeed, the practice of contemporary health governance is coextensive with the practice of health promotion. I conclude by pointing out that critiques of health equity practices have tended to rely far too heavily on hypothetical problems, leaving health equity deliberations troublingly disconnected from hard-earned knowledge about population health.

Health equity is built into population health science

The proper roles of health equity values in population health science are a matter of debate related to Chapter 4's dispute over the "boundary problem" and broad vs. narrow models of public health. Narrow models of public health seek to restrict public health experts from overstepping their professional remit (e.g., by stepping into the contentious social disputes over economic inequality or gun control). This is partially rooted in concerns about what practical effects might happen if public health experts go outside their traditional roles in managing vaccination programs, acting as agents of the state in carrying out local health monitoring, etc. A narrow model of public health restricts public health professionals from taking on the underlying social injustices that cause ill health. That is, the narrow model invites public health expertise into the process of addressing childhood undernutrition, but rejects the proposal that public health professionals have vital roles in social debates about the economic inequalities that cause children to go hungry, since questions about economic policy reform "contain evaluative components which it is not the job of any epidemiologist to answer" (Broadbent 2013: 148). Broadbent offers this strict position while still acknowledging there are normative goals built into epidemiology, a discipline seeking to "improve population health" (Broadbent 2013: 17). Stephen Holland agrees that epidemiology has a "dual aspect" as both a science and an ethically weighty public health practice (Holland 2015). He accordingly allows that some situations require epidemiologists to serve as advocates, such as if their potentially health-enhancing findings were not adequately understood by the public (Holland 2015: 104). He insists, though, that there is no "general duty" to serve as an advocate since "first and foremost, their job is to secure scientific data" (Holland 2015: 105).

While Broadbent and Holland differ somewhat in how comfortable they are with public health experts involving themselves in various ethical disputes, they share the assumption that we can effectively split the fact-gathering practices of the profession from the ethical considerations of the profession. Obviously, nobody is advocating for epidemiologists to unilaterally dictate the ethically superior solution to health-related policy reforms. Rather, there is a long tradition of trying to keep scientists constrained to the jobs of describers or evaluators, chastising them when they begin doing the job of advocate (Pielke 2007).

The more basic question is whether ethical/equity matters can be peeled away from the science and practice of population health in the first place. The population health consequences of assuming we can split the science this way become clear in the fight over whether "population health has an intrinsically distributive dimension" (Reid 2016: 27). As illustrated by Lynette Reid (Reid 2016), John Coggon worries that Marcel Verweij and Angus Dawson are misguided in their understanding of whether inequality can be called a public health harm per se (Verweij and Dawson 2009). Coggon resists Verweij and Dawson's contention that two hypothetical populations could have the same mean health (e.g., the same average life expectancy), but that one of the populations could be judged to have worse public health simply because it has a wider spread of variation—that is, the idea that wide health inequality is judged as a public health detriment in itself (Coggon 2012). Such a view of inequality worries Coggon.

> It seems hard for this not to entail wider claims about the normative value of equity in society, and then to fall into a claim about better versus worse societies, disguised as a more morally neutral claim about healthier versus less healthy societies.
>
> (Coggon 2012: 42)

I understand Coggon's concern about covert values influencing population health assessments—what Pielke calls "stealth issue advocacy" (Pielke 2007). Coggon acknowledges, "the point of public health is to protect and enhance the health of populations" (Coggon 2012: 121), nevertheless, he wishes to keep distribution/variation/inequality considerations out of such health assessments.[1]

Coggon's critique is wrong to assert that distribution/equity considerations are something improperly tacked on to the process of health assessment, or at least in the case of population health science. Population health science is inherently concerned with the distribution of health; explicit concern for the *distribution* of health outcomes is built into definitions of population health and population health science (Kindig 2007; Keyes and Galea 2016; Nash et al. 2016; Diez Roux 2016). An average health outcome (e.g., average life expectancy in Ghana) is a highly compressed data point. Population health science is wise to demote average health's influence by promoting health *distribution* as a primary concern: "population health is defined as health outcomes and their distribution in a population" (Kindig 2007: 141). Two societies with equal mean health in some metric, but different distributions around that mean, are immensely different when viewed from a scientific perspective that explicitly takes distribution to be a primary subject of concern. We can dispute how much worse it is to have distribution A vs. distribution B. But, an assumption that two societies are objectively scientifically equivalent because of having the same mean—prior to any equity and distribution-based value judgments we heap on top of the objective data—is incompatible with population health science. As Katikireddi and I put it in a 2015 article: "It is widely accepted that a fundamental purpose of public health is ameliorating unacceptable health inequalities or health disparities" (Katikireddi and Valles 2015: e36). Health equity is woven into the fabric of population health science and arguably most contemporary conceptions of public health science—the two can be hard to distinguish (DeSalvo et al. 2016; Diez Roux 2016).

Chapter 2 surveys how empirical evidence has shaped population health science's ethical norms, and the relationship works in the opposite direction too. Philosophically, once an ethical value is established in the population health science community, or any scientific community, it then serves to guide and reinforce future evidence collection and assessment—this is not a bad thing (Reiss 2015). Under his self-described pragmatist analysis of the nature of scientific evidence in general, Reiss coincidentally uses a population health example as an illustration—smoking–lung cancer research (Reiss 2015). The public health community of 1950s smoking–cancer researchers had a "widely shared norm that public health should address the fundamental causes of disease and aim to prevent adverse health outcomes" (Reiss 2015: 357). This shared norm helped the community to resolve the epistemic/evidentiary challenge of deciding when there was sufficient evidence to firmly declare that smoking causes lung cancer; the graveness of the health harms clearly outweighed the risks of perhaps being wrong and harming the tobacco industry (Reiss 2015). Not only does evidence legitimately guide the ethical values of scientific communities, but also ethical values can legitimately guide the evidence.

The tight interconnectedness of evidentiary and ethical aspects of science has been described in a variety of ways. For example, Katikireddi and I argue that at least some complex research design questions in public health practice require explicit attention to the dynamic interrelations between ethical issues and epistemic/evidentiary issues—calling for "coupled ethical-epistemic analysis" (Katikireddi and Valles 2015). For example, measurement systems for socioeconomic deprivation have the risk of stigmatizing socioeconomically heterogeneous neighborhoods as "deprived" (an epistemic decision with ethical consequences). That ethical problem of stigma can then, in turn, lead to community members distrusting the researchers or policymakers who stigmatized their neighborhoods, which threatens to impede future cooperation during follow-up research on that population (Katikireddi and Valles 2015).

Taking a general position on the nature of science, philosopher of science Sharyn Clough argues that the line between evidence and values is not so stark as we typically imagine. She critiques those who, in the name of protecting scientific objectivity, wish to put strict limitations on the roles that can be played by ethical value judgments in scientific practice:

> this construal presumes the representationalist view that the empirical data and our feminist political values emanate from two metaphysically separate spheres—the first from the objective, external world; the second from the subjective, internal mind (or minds).

> (Clough 2003: 115)

By contrast, Clough points out that evidential judgments and value judgments are fully connected within each person's "web of belief" (Clough 2003: 117). As she puts it, "our scientific theories and our beliefs about oppression and justice are not merely relative to our conceptual schemes; they are justified by the evidence and they are true" (Clough 2003: 127).

This section of the chapter comes first because it is crucial to enter into the health equity disputes only after recognizing that population health evidence and population health ethics are so tightly intertwined in population health science that we cannot separate the two. Population health science's ethical commitments to equity, and the nuances therein, are founded on a long series of experiences in health practice. This is precisely what is shown in Chapter 2's history of population health science, in which a central role was played by the accumulation of empirical data that brazen social injustices (poverty, etc.) serve as powerful (social) determinants of health. Ward et al.—like Reiss and Clough—try to get at the practical consequences by drawing on pragmatist philosophy. They insist that we need to recognize the normative and descriptive aspects of health inequalities, and that productive social dialogue about these requires explicitly discussing the rationales used in making normative and descriptive judgments (Ward et al. 2013). Whatever decision-making processes are adopted in each context, must include transparency and accountability. Similarly, I agree with Kjellsson et al. that the problem is not so much that values influence public health practice at all, but that the influence can be both subtle and manipulative. They show how one's choice of which specific relative measures to use in mortality rate calculations can make a given population appear more or less healthy (Kjellsson et al. 2015). Crucially, in their account of the problem, Kjellsson et al. illustrate their point with a combination of theoretical discussion, a hypothetical mathematical case, and most importantly examples of how the issues play out in real world practice (analyzing health disparities between European nations). Philosophical disputes over health equity are prone to becoming untethered from our empirical knowledge, to the detriment of health equity discourse. Again, we cannot simply split apart the science and the ethics of population health, and we certainly ought not lose sight of the empirical data available to us.

The (real and imagined) consequences of an ambiguous understanding of "health equity"

There is a diverse array of theoretical positions on what health equity is, and what its moral roots are. In this chapter, I am not interested in trying to offer another competitor position to the list of options. I am instead interested in challenging some key assumptions in these philosophical debates: (1) that the theoretical aspects of health equity debates must be settled, lest bad practical consequences ensue (challenged in this section); and (2) these debates must properly resolve in a single consensus position (challenged in the next section). What sort of a problem—and how large of a problem—is it for population health equity to have lingering ambiguities in its meaning and fundamental moral foundations? I have devoted a substantial portion of my career to analyzing the perils of ambiguous concepts in population health ("trait," "race," "normal," etc.) (Valles 2012a, 2012b, 2013, 2016a). Coming from that position, I still caution against the assumption that conceptual ambiguities or disputes automatically delegitimize applications of the embattled concepts.

I am troubled by the meta-philosophical assumption that ambiguous or debated moral conceptual foundations for policies delegitimize work done on top of those foundations. For example, Preda and Voigt philosophically critique Marmot's WHO *Closing the Gap* report (Commission on Social Determinants of Health 2008) for having inadequate foundations for its health equity efforts, but identify no specific policy proposals in the report that actually need to be rejected (Preda and Voigt 2015). Goldberg's commentary on Preda and Voigt's critique is more sympathetic toward population health practitioners, but still criticizes their inattention: "the ... energy and teamwork for which public health practitioners are rightly renowned must be leveraged in service of the very idea of health equity" (Goldberg 2015: S12). Neither text seems to question the tacit assumption that theoretical weakness dooms practical applications.

Instead of critiquing actual proposals from the WHO Social Determinants report, Preda and Voigt point out that reducing the social determinants of smoking is probably insufficient to eliminate smoking disparities (Preda and Voigt 2015). This is not so shocking since nicotine is addictive. In an analogous theoretical critique, Goldberg points out that the population health literature's advocacy of interventions to reduce avoidable disparities runs into an intuitive exception in the case of sex disparities in prostate cancer rates (Goldberg 2015). In the real world, who is advocating that we *should* be addressing sex disparities in prostate cancer rates?

I don't dispute the existence of ambiguous concepts and challenging cases, but the key philosophical question is how philosophers, population health professionals, and policymakers should all proceed in light of this. Goldberg is the most effective philosopher advocate of broad models of population health (Chapter 4), and defends health equity scholarship as an ongoing enterprise. But he still claims, "what passes for normative recommendations in SDOH policy discourse fails," because it simplistically leaps from "the social epidemiologic evidence to normative conclusions without attending to any of the intervening steps in the argument" (Goldberg 2015: 58–59). He later (Goldberg 2016) cites Venkatapuram's incisive critiques of these ambiguities. Yet, Venkatapuram offers a more productive way of proceeding in light of disputes about health equity. In fact, Marmot writes the introduction to Venkatapuram's book, seeing it as providing "better articulation of philosophical underpinnings" left unsaid in the "Closing the Gap" report (Venkatapuram 2011). Marmot's Commission had argued:

> The right to the highest attainable standard of health is enshrined in the Constitution of the [World Health Organization] and numerous international treaties. But the degree to which these rights are met from one place to another around the world is glaringly unequal. Social injustice is killing people on a grand scale.
>
> (Commission on Social Determinants of Health 2008: 26)

After hearing subsequent critiques, Marmot countered that Venkatapuram's account suffices as a "theoretical justification" for those working in applied health equity:

Every human being has a moral entitlement to a capability to be healthy ... and to a level that is commensurate with equal human dignity in the contemporary world.

(Venkatapuram 2011)

There are other viable operational definitions available, as well. Preda and Voigt declare they are dissatisfied with Margaret Whitehead's influential operational definition of health equity (Preda and Voigt 2015):

Equity in health implies that ideally everyone should have a fair opportunity to attain their full health potential and, more pragmatically, that no one should be disadvantaged from achieving this potential, if it can be avoided.

(Whitehead 1990)

It should be noted that this definition is something Whitehead derives from interpretation of previous WHO work, and writes into a WHO report for the purpose of guiding future WHO work, so it is as much a description of what WHO *does* believe as a normative proposal of what it *should* believe (Whitehead 1990: 7). There is unquestionably a need for continuing debate over these varying accounts of health equity and its moral foundation—in fact, Whitehead explicitly says this (Whitehead 1990: 3). My worry here is that critics in the philosophy of health equity community have not established what would qualify as a sufficiently rigorous operational definition and philosophical foundation for applied health equity work.

I contend that settling on a very specific health equity principle (e.g., Whitehead's or Venkatapuram's) and a corresponding ethical justification are neither a necessary nor a sufficient means for a community to sort out its health justice priorities. As much as it pains philosophers to admit it, most people live their entire lives without developing an informed stance on the philosophical foundations of their ethical commitments, including the nature of social justice (in health or other areas of life). But, ethical conduct does not seem to primarily hinge on the degree to which one scrutinizes and tweaks basic philosophical principles. Indeed, (very limited) experimental evidence indicates that professional ethicists do not demonstrate any special ability to lead lives consistent with their finely tuned ethical stances (Schwitzgebel and Rust 2014). This book is written in the spirit of a belief that philosophy can, despite this, contribute substantially to the improved theory and practice of population health science. I just lack faith in the power of forming a public consensus on ethical key terms as a means of securing health justice in the world.

The premise that the public (or perhaps just health professionals) ought to settle on and rally around one specific health equity principle and one set of moral foundations for those principles seems like a recipe for predictable failure in a world that is increasingly defined by migration and multicultural coexistence. Informed dialogue has utterly failed to generate consensus even within the community of professional philosophers of public health, so I am baffled by the apparent assumption that population health practitioners or policymakers ought to reach such a consensus. Why expect communities of non-ethicists to be any more ethically concordant than professional ethicists? Perhaps my pluralist commitments have prevented me from understanding the appeal of reaching consensus in ethical discourse.

Conceptions of "health equity" have practical limitations, similar to the ones that Sen identifies for the related concept "justice." He warns that pursuing an idealized understanding of the nature of justice—"any answer to the grand question 'What is a just society?'"—is "neither necessary nor sufficient" for helping us to make the world a more just place. On the other hand, we can have an understanding of how to make the world *more* just "without containing—or entailing—an answer to the question" of what ideally defines a just society (Sen 2006: 236–237). We don't need to have an immaculate definition of justice to make the world more just, and we can develop a "thoroughly usable" plan for promoting justice without ever settling on such a definition (Sen 2006: 236). In a similar line of argument, Schwartz argues the problem of defining health should not be about concept analysis of health's meaning, but more about concept "explication." In the tradition of Carnap and Quine: we should be most of all concerned with adjusting health/disease concepts *more illuminating and/or more useful* (Schwartz 2014). Lemoine (2013) and Griffiths and Matthewson (2016) make similar points about philosophy of medicine's excessive attention to analyzing the boundaries of health/disease concepts. So it is for health equity. We can make progress on ameliorating the world's appallingly inequitable health patterns without first (or perhaps ever) deciding "What *is* an equitably healthy society?" Debates about the nature of health equity are good, but what we pressingly need are decision-making processes for determining what constitutes the best means of addressing health equity problems, from the local level through the global level.

Equitable health promotion and health governance

As Keyes and Galea describe in their account of population health science, the question is not *whether* equitable distribution of health is an intrinsic part of population health science (the discipline has equity concerns built into its foundations), but *who* will have control over setting and assessing the equity goals and trade-offs of population health. I agree.

> Population health scientists have a moral obligation to address inequalities as they arise from inequities in the distribution of resources ... Understanding who sets the goals and whether those goals are optimal for maximizing population health remains, perhaps, the most important job of a population health scientist.
>
> (Keyes and Galea 2016: 139)

I do not pretend to have the formula for what constitutes good health governance. Not only is that far more ambitious a goal than can be achieved in a single section of a single chapter, but good governance will be significantly locally contingent in many of its details, and even its general contours are hazy and subject to dispute (Levi-Faur 2012). McHugh lucidly illustrates the local contingency of health knowledge and pragmatic action in the detailed case studies of health governance and equity in her book (McHugh 2015).

In the case of health governance, Ilona Kickbusch, who was a driving force behind the Ottawa Charter featured in Chapter 2 (World Health Organization 1986), frames health governance as something that does and should co-evolve with our theoretical and empirical understandings of health and disease (Kickbusch 2007). Her history of the key recent developments that affected current health governance ideology overlaps partly with the events I feature in Chapter 2's account of the origins of population health science and the gradual understanding of health as a multidimensional social phenomenon: the Lalonde Report (Lalonde 1974) and the Ottawa Charter (World Health Organization 1986).

Kickbusch extracts the lesson that contemporary health governance is best understood as *coextensive* with health promotion, which makes health governance as perplexing and as poorly understood as health promotion in general (Kickbusch 2007). What is clear though, on her account, is that health governance must accordingly be as diffuse as the agents that influence health and the affected stakeholders. It turns out to be the case that health's causes and effects are both fully interwoven in the fabric of social life (Kickbusch 2007). She cites the example of smoking governance, which is not just a matter of which laws are made (or whether such laws balance public good and individual liberty—a classic public health ethics concern), but no less a matter of how legal norms and cultural norms are taken up by actors, such as restaurant staff (the people who actually implement regulations), and by the citizens whose culture accepts or rejects smoking norms, either pulling the governance process forward, or lagging behind it (Kickbusch 2007).

I second Kickbusch's plea for health governance discourse to turn attention to the "settings of everyday life" (Kickbusch 2007: 157). That has hopefully been clear throughout this book. After Chapter 2's positioning of the Ottawa Charter as a milestone in the development of understandings of health as social, Chapter 3 argues that health should be defined as a life course trajectory of complete well-being in social context; Chapter 4 elaborates that these diffuse everyday settings require a broad model of health promotion (stretching into all corners of social life); Chapter 5 argues that this synchronizes with a need to address the underlying social factors that drive health disparities. Addressing health when it is so deeply connected to social life also requires knowledge that reflects such. Kickbusch and Gleicher elaborate on this in a 2012 WHO report, "Governance for health in the 21st century" (Kickbusch and Gleicher 2012).

> successful governance for health requires co-production as well as the involvement and cooperation of citizens, consumers and patients. As governance becomes more widely diffused throughout society, working directly with the public can strengthen transparency and accountability.
>
> (Kickbusch and Gleicher 2012: x)

Chapter 8 will elaborate on this point, along with their related claim about health epistemology, that is, our conception of health knowledge and expertise: "co-production of health implies co-production of knowledge. If governance for health is to be effective, it must be participatory and include but transcend expert opinion" (Kickbusch and Gleicher 2012: 14).

To summarize, health is socially produced in everyday life and must be promoted accordingly (World Health Organization 1986). Health governance is health promotion, but the right means of undertaking health promotion remains hazy, spread across all areas of daily life in society, and is locally contingent (Kickbusch 2007; McHugh 2015). Finally, the knowledge we need to work on health promotion must be co-produced by a diverse group of credentialed experts, alongside laypeople (Kickbusch and Gleicher 2012).

Insofar as health governance *is* health promotion, nobody knows how to govern health any more than they know how to promote it. Health promotion is not a total mystery, but so much about it remains unknown—even the field of population health science is quite young. But, based on the lessons of the preceding chapters, I offer the following guidance for how to make progress-developing processes for health governance, including health equity decision-making processes:

1   Health governance needs to target its efforts to every corner of social life, because health is fully integrated into social life (see Chapter 2). Health *is* social well-being (see Chapter 3), and health governance will be needlessly hampered if it cordons off certain problems or domains as not health matters (see Chapter 4).
2   Health governance should give special attention to the "fundamental" and "upstream" social/environmental causes that serve as drivers of a huge range of proximate health/disease causes (see Chapter 5).
3   Health governance decision makers should carefully attend to how health benefits and detriments accrue to the total population and subpopulations therein. In Chapter 6, I offer specific guidance on how to do this.
4   The upcoming Chapter 8 will further argue why health promotion—and hence health governance—should be characterized by humble and non-hierarchical collaborations between different disciplines and sectors of society, none of whom can claim they have the overarching expertise needed to promote health. Different credentialed experts and un-credentialed laypeople have knowledge of different segments of the tapestry of social life and health/well-being therein.

As indicated in item (4), humility will be a subject of the next chapter, but for the purpose of this chapter, it is fitting to begin that discussion by addressing my own profession's need to demonstrate humility.

Hypothetical problems' outsized influence in population health equity deliberations

I fully endorse calls for population health science professionals to be cautious and aware of their own limitations when they render health equity judgments. That said, I similarly ask that philosophers of population health (broadly construed) be cautious and aware of their own limitations when they render judgments about population health scientists' practices. Chapter 8 will further elaborate on this point, and suffice to say here that the need for humility applies to all parties involved in the massive joint venture of improving populations' health. Philosophy's role in population health is not as gatekeeper or arbiter of the good. That is one of the reasons why this book on philosophy of population health tends to begin its recommendations for what population health experts ought to do by looking at what they are already doing and proceeding from there. Population health scientists are, as a whole, technically competent, equity-minded, and characterized by the sort of non-doctrinaire and pragmatic open-mindedness that I admire in health professionals. In this context, I urge philosophers of population health equity to stay grounded in existing empirical knowledge of population health science during the debates over health equity. Health equity debates all too often elevate speculative hypothetical problems over specific concrete ones.

Take, for instance, the hypothetical problem of "leveling down," which worries that adopting the wrong definition of equity could make it hypothetically possible for us to achieve greater equity by harming those who are currently better off, when we would surely prefer to raise up those who are now most disadvantaged (Parfit 1997; Broome 2002; Eyal 2013). A health equity concept may look promising, but can it pass the test of the leveling down problem by reliably blocking monstrous hypothetical policymakers from achieving health equity by harming those who are best off? The leveling down problem has received a degree of attention that is more commensurate with its intellectual intrigue than its practical repercussions. It may be an important philosophy problem—many philosophers contend that it is such, and it is their disciplinary prerogative to make that designation—but debate over predominantly hypothetical problems translates to a weak justification for worrying about leveling down as a health equity problem in the world.

The leveling down problem has its own section and section editor in the Phil-Papers archive, and appears in an edited volume on the 100 most important Western Philosophy problems (Saunders 2011). It is an intriguing idea. Kurt Vonnegut piqued science fiction readers' interest by imagining a world where health inequities are resolved by burdening the healthy with literal weights tied around their bodies. The late conservative icon, US Supreme Court Justice Scalia used Vonnegut's short story in his dissent against a landmark ruling that affirmed the legal rights of the disabled (Scalia 2001). Harder to find are actual concrete instances of the leveling down problem hurting people—even in the literature on the population health dimensions of it (Brock 2012).

Leveling down is not a pseudo-problem—Nir Eyal has shown that it comes up in a policy that rejects organ donations from racist donors who would insist on specifying that their donations only go to White patients (Eyal 2013). The strange case of proactive racist organ donors is a step up in practical significance from Derek Parfit's fascinating original formulation of the problem, which cites only hypothetical examples, including a discussion of hypothetical policies for blinding the sighted or surgically stealing their eyes to give to the blind(!) (Parfit 1997). Similarly, Temkin's famous paper on the subject brushes up against a concrete case by discussing whether he ought to give money to one of his daughters over the other, but quickly turns into a fantastical scenario in which one daughter finds a discarded $20 bill on the street every week, and has a life that is in every single respect slightly better than her sibling's (Temkin 2003). It all makes for perfectly good fodder for philosophers and science fiction writers (and, apparently, legal jurists like Scalia, looking to justify a disregard for the disabled).

Hypothetical debates that are loosely tethered to our empirical knowledge can serve as harmful distractions, and must be used carefully. There is great value in exploring hypothetical problems, but it raises red flags when scholarly presentations of hypothetical problems lack accompanying evidence that such problems have occurred, do occur, or are have a serious risk of occurring in the real world. A particularly poignant illustration comes in the form of an anecdote from Marmot. Nobel laureate health economist Angus Deaton once asked if Marmot would prefer a society with low inequality between social classes but generally poor health for all, or a society with more severe inequality but in which every social class was better off than in the first society. Marmot "rejected both alternatives" and instead argued that there is no empirical reason why one must choose between these two options (Marmot 2004: 245–246). We could have a hypothetical health equity debate wherein we must choose between equally poor health for everyone or a steep gradient that includes excellent health for some and abysmal health for others. But there's no compelling reason for assuming those are the only two options. We face so many hard health equity choices that we ought to be cautious about inventing new problems.

Conclusion

Population health science developed its specific equity commitments and priorities largely as the consequence of new empirical data. The population health framework didn't just develop its methodologies to match practitioners' values, which happened to prioritize social reform. Rather, the historical record in Chapter 2 shows how the process seemed to go more in the opposite causal direction, though, now that those values are established (especially the pursuit of health equity), they can and should guide future collection and assessment of empirical data (Reiss 2015).

There seems to be universal agreement among philosophers and practitioners of public/population health that health equity deliberations must include diligent attention to questions of priority-setting. Where I depart from many of my philosopher colleagues is on the matter of how best to go about moving toward a just set of priorities. I argue that many have been sidetracked by hypothetical problems (rather than concrete ones) and an over-prioritization of debates about the nature and moral underpinnings of health equity. Instead, I argue health promotion and health governance—the two are now more or less coextensive—and health equity priority-setting are all best advanced by fostering participatory and substantially locally driven processes. These processes should be driven not by academic debates over the single right moral theory or equity concept, but rather by careful construction of participatory processes that empower the affected populations to take the lead in directing their own health.

Chapter 8 will proceed to show how the need to engage with communities in designing interventions requires reconceptualizing the relationships between interdisciplinary population health experts and lay individuals/groups from the populations being served. Health promotion cannot be airdropped from foreign aid cargo planes, nor can equitable health interventions be designed by distant experts. This has many implications for the future of population health science. First, though, this chapter will conclude with a case study illustrating its points, the case of the global research effort to investigate racism and racial health disparities.

Case study: investigating racism and racial health disparities

The international interdisciplinary research community of scholars of racial and ethnic health disparities is a model of health equity practice, due to its rigorous theoretical and methodological disputes balanced with a track record of fruitful cooperation. This case study illustrates how the common ethical goal of ameliorating racism is able to hold together the research community despite their disparate views about the nature of equity and other core concepts such as the nature of race.

Equity concerns are built into the population health science of racial health disparities. This is perhaps most vividly illustrated in Mir et al.'s structured consensus-building exercise with a group of international experts on race/ ethnicity and health. The resulting consensus statement consists of only ten items, the first of which announces:

> The purpose of research on ethnicity and health should be for the well-being and betterment of populations being studied and equity should be the guiding ethical principle.
>
> (Mir et al. 2013: 508)

This statement is a bold declaration of the proper *goals* of research on racial/ ethnic minority populations' health, not just the typical loose constraints offered by guidelines on the "responsible conduct of research" (Tuana 2010). The consensus statement does not even leave room for research done in the spirit of truth/knowledge as an end in itself. Instead, as I have explained in previous work, it demands that race research has the goal of ameliorating racism, and this is indeed the proper ethical resolution to the question of whether/how to use race concepts in health research (Valles 2016b). The guidelines (rightly) even cut off research designed to use insights from one group for the sole purpose of bene-fitting another group (Valles 2016a). Research on marginalized racial or ethnic groups inevitably creates risks for those groups—any evidence of good health can serve as an excuse to further deprive the population of social resources and evidence of poor health can serve as a confirmation of stigma and perceived inferiority (Valles 2016a: 143). In this context of ever-present risk of harm to the population being studied, research must remain faithfully aimed at benefits making the research worth the risks (Valles 2016a). Based on the above commit-ment to the purpose of minority health research, seven other Principles address the general contours of equity-serving work: the ethical mandate to address ethnic health disparities, close attention to intersectional dynamics between vari-eties of difference, promotion of participatory research methods, and exhorta-tions to analyze the social and environmental determinants of "inequalities" and "disadvantage" (Mir et al. 2013: 508; see Table 7.1).

Not having a full definition of health equity does not prevent scholars of racial and ethnic health disparities from doing good work. As noted above, the community disagrees about the meaning of race and ethnicity (Modood et al. 2002; Smith 2002; Cohn 2006; Cho 2006; Valles 2016b), but this does not prevent them from using the terms productively in applied research. The Leeds Consensus itself proclaims the goal of pursuing "equity" but declines to commit to a detailed definition of it (Mir et al. 2013: 508). Along similar lines, the new journal *Health Equity*, devoted to racial and ethnic health disparities among other topics, declares that it "was founded to deliver authoritative, peer-reviewed, information and contribute to the empowerment of communities to identify and solve pervasive problems related to health and wellness" (Núñez and Schilling 2017: 1)—none of these concrete goals requires reaching a con-sensus on the question of what exactly constitutes equitable health between different racial and ethnic groups.

Health governance and health promotion are inseparable in applied popula-tion health science. And health promotion must, for the reasons spelled out above, tend to health causes and effects in their natural habitats: the "settings of everyday life" (Kickbusch 2007: 157). A fitting example of this comes from the University of Edinburgh Centre for Population Health Sciences' Edinburgh Ethnicity, Migration, and Health Research Group, which I briefly joined as a vis-iting scholar, a group that includes Raj Bhopal (my former co-author) and Aziz Sheikh, who worked on the Leeds Consensus project. Bhopal and Sheikh are two of the leaders of an illustrative health equity project called Prevention of Diabetes of South Asians—PODOSA (Bhopal et al. 2014; Morrison et al. 2014). The project aims to better understand, and craft interventions for, the exception-ally high rates of diabetes among (heterogeneous) ethnic South Asians living in the UK. To understand why these populations were burdened by this disparate

Table 7.1 The Leeds Consensus Principles for research on ethnicity and health.

Importance and purpose

1 Ethnicity is often associated with disadvantage and ill health. Researchers consequently have both a professional and ethical responsibility to incorporate evidence on ethnicity into their work and recommendations.

2 The purpose of research on ethnicity and health should be for the well-being and betterment of populations being studied and equity should be the guiding ethical principle. Researchers must be alert to the dangers of discriminatory thinking and behavior and guard against actual and potential harm resulting from their research.

Framing and focus

3 It is important to be explicit about the assumptions and theories that underlie research on ethnicity and health.

4 There is a need for research to, where appropriate, examine diversity within ethnic groups and avoid homogenization. For example, age, gender, religion, education, socioeconomic position, geography, or time of migration may all impact on the generation of ethnic health inequalities. Investigation of ethnic health inequalities should pay due regard to the ways in which ethnicity intersects with other forms of difference in order to understand how and why it may be relevant.

5 There is a need to improve the participation of minority ethnic communities in all stages of the research process. Appropriate participation should be defined by these communities, then promoted by researchers and statutory agencies and resourced by funding bodies.

Data collection and analysis

6 The use of ethnic categories and labels should be meaningful in relation to the particular experiences and outcomes being explored.

7 Census categories are often useful for exposing disadvantage, but additional measures may be needed to explore the processes through which disadvantage is created.

8 Analysis of health inequalities should pay attention to the social context in which ethnic differences in health outcomes are measured and health behaviors occur.

Future priorities

9 There is a need to focus on intervention studies that help identify effective ways of reducing inequalities.

10. More research is needed on appropriate models for involving minority ethnic communities throughout the research process. For example, models for community capacity-building, empowerment, representativeness, and continuity of engagement.

Source: Mir et al. 2013: 508.

disease rate, the project had to look closely at populations' social lives. For example, researchers needed to learn who actually shops for food and cooks family meals, and listen to participants' reports of which social pressures made them more or less likely to adhere to a modified diet plan (Morrison et al. 2014). It turns out that complex social dynamics come into play, such as, a family whose traditional Indo-Pakistani dishes were chosen and prepared with children's palates and cultural identities in mind, since such food (in the UK) is always in competition with "food like from McDonald's" (Morrison et al. 2014).

As illustrated in the PODOSA example, one of the biggest challenges for racial/ethnic health disparities health researchers has been the crafting of effective methods for carrying out their interests in identifying and intervening upon the health inequities arising out of social and environmental determinants in everyday life. Two of the ten Leeds Consensus Principles stress the importance of participatory research processes. One of the principles states outright that minority communities must be involved in all stages of research. Even the judgment of what qualifies as sufficient community participation is a decision that must be delegated to the community, and then researchers, according to the Principle, must advocate for that decision. Another Principle calls for further refinement:

> More research is needed on appropriate models for involving minority ethnic communities throughout the research process. For example, models for community capacity building, empowerment, representativeness and continuity of engagement.
>
> (Mir et al. 2013: 508)

This repeats similar points by the Commission on Social Determinants of Health (Commission on Social Determinants of Health 2008), by Ranco et al. (cited in the Chapter 2 case study of Standing Rock Sioux health) (Ranco et al. 2011), and also by Australian government (cited in the Chapter 3 case study of Aboriginal Australian health) (Government of Western Australia Department of Health 2015). The PODOSA project worked within such an ambitious participatory ideal by making inclusivity and the formation of trusting relationships part of the project strategy from its inception (Douglas et al. 2011). Tellingly, efforts to recruit participants by working with healthcare providers was largely unsuccessful, but found success through "community orientated, personal approaches for recruitment" such as reaching out to community leaders and visiting mosques.

The racial health disparities research community has demonstrated an admirable commitment to following the empirical data wherever it leads, and adjusting equity priorities accordingly. There have been shifts also in the conceptualizing and measurement of racism; among other shifts, structural racism (the racism embedded in social structures, broadly construed) is getting wider use (Rudolph et al. 2013). And it is only relatively recently that attention has been turning to racism as a direct cause in its own right (Krieger 2003). However, the data collection, compilation, synthesis of health effects from racism's heterogeneous pathways (from the stress of micro-aggressions to reduced access to social services) has proven exceptionally difficult (Paradies et al. 2015). The community of researchers specializing in racial and ethnic health disparities did work, do work, and will continue working toward health equity, unhampered by ambiguities in the precise meaning of equity, but carefully attending to the nuances of applied health promotion/governance. They don't agree on everything, but they agree on more than enough to keep them busy for decades to come.

Note

1 This goal is tied to his position that population health is merely the sum of its individual members' health. As illustrated in Chapter 3, citing Onyebuchi Arah's work, my definition of health addresses Coggon's worry that individual health and population health could be incommensurable sorts of things. Chapter 3 argues that the two levels of health are dynamically linked through the social and temporal nature of well-being—that individual health and population health co-develop.

Works cited

Ankeny, R. A. (2003) How history and philosophy of science could save the life of bioethics. *Journal of Medicine and Philosophy* 28, 115–125.

Bhopal, R. S., Douglas, A., Wallia, S., et al. (2014) Effect of a lifestyle intervention on weight change in South Asian individuals in the UK at high risk of type 2 diabetes: A family-cluster randomised controlled trial. *The Lancet Diabetes & Endocrinology* 2, 218–227.

Broadbent, A. (2013) *Philosophy of Epidemiology*. New York: Palgrave Macmillan.

Brock, D. W. (2012) Priority to the Worse Off in Health Care Resource Prioritization. In: Rhodes, R., Battin, M. and Silvers, A. (eds) *Medicine and Social Justice: Essays on the Distribution of Health Care*. Oxford: Oxford University Press, 155–164.

Broome, J. (2002) Fairness, Goodness and Levelling Down. In: Murray, C. J. L., Salomon, J. A., Mathers, C. D., et al. (eds) *Summary Measures of Population Health: Concepts, Ethics, Measurement and Applications*. Geneva: World Health Organization, 135–137.

Cho, M. K. (2006) Racial and ethnic categories in biomedical research: There is no baby in the bathwater. *Journal of Law, Medicine and Ethics* 34, 497–499.

Clough, S. (2003) *Beyond Epistemology: A Pragmatist Approach to Feminist Science Studies*. New York: Rowman and Littlefield, Inc.

Coggon, J. (2012) *What Makes Health Public? A Critical Evaluation of Moral, Legal, and Political Claims in Public Health*. New York: Cambridge University Press.

Cohn, J. N. (2006) The use of race and ethnicity in medicine: Lessons from the African-American Heart Failure Trial. *Journal of Law, Medicine and Ethics* 34, 552–554.

Commission on Social Determinants of Health. (2008) Closing the Gap in a Generation: Health Equity Through Action on the Social Determinants of Health. Geneva: World Health Organization.

Daniels, N. (2008) *Just Health: Meeting Health Needs Fairly*. New York: Cambridge University Press.

DeSalvo, K. B., O'Carroll, P. W., Koo, D., et al. (2016) Public health 3.0: Time for an upgrade. *American Journal of Public Health* 106, 621–622.

Diez Roux, A. V. (2016) On the distinction—or lack of distinction—between population health and public health. *American Journal of Public Health* 106, 619–620.

Douglas, A., Bhopal, R. S., Bhopal, R., et al. (2011) Recruiting South Asians to a lifestyle intervention trial: Experiences and lessons from PODOSA (Prevention of Diabetes & Obesity in South Asians). *Trials* 12, 220.

Eyal, N. (2013) Leveling Down Health. In: Eyal, N., Hurst, S. A., Norheim, O. F., et al. (eds) *Inequalities in Health: Concepts, Measures, and Ethics*. Oxford: Oxford University Press, 197–213.

Goldberg, D. (2015) The naturalistic fallacy in ethical discourse on the social determinants of health. *The American Journal of Bioethics* 15, 58–60.

Goldberg, D. (2016) On the very idea of health equity. *Journal of Public Health Management and Practice* 22, S11–S12.

Government of Western Australia Department of Health. (2015) WA Aboriginal Health and Wellbeing Framework 2015–2030. http://ww2.health.wa.gov.au/Improving-WA-Health/About-Aboriginal-Health/WA-Aboriginal-Health-and-Wellbeing-Framework-2015-2030: Department of Health.

Griffiths, P. E. and Matthewson, J. (2016) Evolution, dysfunction, and disease: A reappraisal. *The British Journal for the Philosophy of Science*. Available at: https://doi.org/10.1093/bjps/axw021.

Holland, S. (2015) *Public Health Ethics*. Malden, MA: Polity Press.

Katikireddi, S. V. and Valles, S. A. (2015) Coupled ethical-epistemic analysis of public health research and practice: Categorizing variables to improve population health and equity. *American Journal of Public Health* 105, e36–e42.

Keyes, K. M. and Galea, S. (2016) *Population Health Science*. New York: Oxford University Press.

Kickbusch, I. (2007) Health governance: The health society. In McQueen, D. V. and Kickbusch, I. (eds) *Health and Modernity*. New York: Springer, 144–161.

Kickbusch, I. and Gleicher, D. (2012) Governance for Health in the 21st Century. Copenhagen: World Health Organization Regional Office for Europe.

Kindig, D. A. (2007) Understanding population health terminology. *Milbank Quarterly* 85, 139–161.

Kjellsson, G., Gerdtham, U.-G. and Petrie, D. (2015) Lies, damned lies, and health inequality measurements: Understanding the value judgments. *Epidemiology* 26, 673–680.

Krieger, N. (2003) Does racism harm health? Did child abuse exist before 1962? On explicit questions, critical science, and current controversies: An ecosocial perspective. *American Journal of Public Health* 93, 194–199.

Lalonde, M. (1974) *A New Perspective on the Health of Canadians*. Ottawa, Canada: Health and Welfare Canada.

Lemoine, M. (2013) Defining disease beyond conceptual analysis: An analysis of conceptual analysis in philosophy of medicine. *Theoretical Medicine and Bioethics* 34, 309–325.

Levi-Faur, D. (2012) *The Oxford Handbook of Governance*. Oxford: Oxford University Press.

Marmot, M. (2004) *The Status Syndrome: How Social Standing Affects Our Health and Longevity*. New York: Henry Holt and Company.

McHugh, N. A. (2015) *The Limits of Knowledge: Generating Pragmatist Feminist Cases for Situated Knowing*. Albany, NY: SUNY Press.

Mir, G., Salway, S., Kai, J., et al. (2013) Principles for research on ethnicity and health: the Leeds Consensus Statement. *The European Journal of Public Health* 23, 504–510.

Modood, T., Berthoud, R. and Nazroo, J. (2002) "Race," racism and ethnicity: A response to Ken Smith. *Sociology* 36, 419–427.

Morrison, Z., Douglas, A., Bhopal, R. and Sheikh, A. (2014) Understanding experiences of participating in a weight loss lifestyle intervention trial: A qualitative evaluation of South Asians at high risk of diabetes. *BMJ Open* 4, e004736.

Nash, D. B., Fabius, R. J., Skoufalos, A., et al. (2016) *Population Health: Creating a Culture of Wellness*. Second ed. Burlington, MA: Jones & Bartlett Learning.

Núñez, A. and Schilling, J. L. (2017) A space to promote intentional thoughtful action. *Health Equity* 1, 1.

Nussbaum, M. C. (2011) *Creating Capabilities: The Human Development Approach.* Cambridge: Belknap Press.

Paradies, Y., Ben, J., Denson, N., et al. (2015) Racism as a determinant of health: A systematic review and meta-analysis. *PloS One* 10, e0138511.

Parfit, D. (1997) Equality and priority. *Ratio* 10, 202–221.

Pielke, R. A. (2007) *The Honest Broker: Making Sense of Science in Policy and Politics.* Cambridge: Cambridge University Press.

Powers, M. and Faden, R. R. (2006) *Social Justice: The Moral Foundations of Public Health and Health Policy.* New York: Oxford University Press.

Preda, A. and Voigt, K. (2015) The social determinants of health: Why should we care? *The American Journal of Bioethics* 15, 25–36.

Ranco, D. J., O'Neill, C. A., Donatuto, J. and Harper, B. L. (2011) Environmental justice, American Indians and the cultural dilemma: Developing environmental management for tribal health and well-being. *Environmental Justice* 4, 221–230.

Reid, L. (2016) Does population health have an intrinsically distributional dimension? *Public Health Ethics* 9, 24–36.

Reiss, J. (2015) A pragmatist theory of evidence. *Philosophy of Science* 82, 341–362.

Rudolph, L., Caplan, J., Ben-Moshe, K. and Dillon, L. (2013) *Health in All Policies: A Guide for State and Local Governments.* Washington, DC: American Public Health Association and Public Health Institute.

Ruger, J. P. (2010) *Health and Social Justice.* Oxford: Oxford University Press.

Saunders, B. (2011) Parfit's Leveling Down Argument against Egalitarianism. In: Bruce, M. and Barbone, S. (eds) *Just the Arguments: 100 of the Most Important Arguments in Western Philosophy.* Malden, MA: Blackwell Publishing, 251–253.

Scalia, A. (2001) PGA Tour, Inc. v. Martin. *532 US 661.* United States Supreme Court.

Schwartz, P. H. (2014) Reframing the disease debate and defending the biostatistical theory. *Journal of Medicine and Philosophy* 39, 572–589.

Schwitzgebel, E. and Rust, J. (2014) The moral behavior of ethics professors: Relationships among self-reported behavior, expressed normative attitude, and directly observed behavior. *Philosophical Psychology* 27, 293–327.

Sen, A. (2006) What do we want from a theory of justice? *Journal of Philosophy* 103, 215–238.

Smith, K. (2002) Some Critical Observations on the Use of the Concept of "Ethnicity." In: Modood, T. et al., *Ethnic Minorities in Britain. Sociology* 36, 399–417.

Temkin, L. S. (2003) Egalitarianism defended. *Ethics* 113, 764–782.

Tuana, N. (2010) Leading with ethics, aiming for policy: New opportunities for philosophy of science. *Synthese* 177, 471–492.

Valles, S. A. (2012a) Heterogeneity of risk within racial groups: A challenge for public health programs. *Preventive Medicine* 55, 405–408.

Valles, S. A. (2012b) Lionel Penrose and the concept of normal variation in human intelligence. *Studies in History and Philosophy of Biological and Biomedical Sciences* 43, 231–289.

Valles, S. A. (2013) Validity and utility in biological traits. *Biological Theory* 8, 93–102.

Valles, S. A. (2016a) The challenges of choosing and explaining a phenomenon in epidemiological research on the "Hispanic Paradox." *Theoretical Medicine and Bioethics* 37, 129–148.

Valles, S. A. (2016b) Race in Medicine. In: Solomon, M., Simon, J. R. and Kincaid, H. (eds) *The Routledge Companion to Philosophy of Medicine.* New York: Routledge, 419–431.

Venkatapuram, S. (2011) *Health Justice: An Argument from the Capabilities Approach.* Malden, MA: Polity Press.

Verweij, M. and Dawson, A. (2009) The Meaning of "Public" in Public Health. In: Dawson, A. and Verweij, M. (eds) *Ethics, Prevention, and Public Health.* Oxford: Oxford University Press, 13–29.

Ward, A., Johnson, P. J. and O'Brien, M. (2013) The normative dimensions of health disparities. *Journal of Health Disparities Research and Practice* 6, 46–61.

Whitehead, M. (1990) *The Concepts and Principles of Equity and Health.* Copenhagen: World Health Organization Regional Office for Europe.

World Health Organization (1986) Ottawa Charter for Health Promotion. Ottawa, ON: World Health Organization.

8 Humility as the way forward for population health, and philosophy thereof

Introduction: a spirit of humility and collaboration

Thanks in large part to the Ottawa Charter, population health science has long recognized the need to redistribute the power and authority concentrated in the healthcare sector—"to share power with other sectors, other disciplines and most importantly with people themselves" (World Health Organization 1986). In articulating a feminist alternative to traditionalist scientific virtues, Longino makes a strong case for adopting "decentralization or diffusion of power" as a scientific virtue in its own right—no less valuable than "accuracy" or "novelty" (Longino 1995: 392). In arguing for community-based participatory research, Freudenberg and Tsui implore that scholars and policy advocates of health promotion need to be just as well versed "in the world of power as in the world of evidence" (Freudenberg and Tsui 2014: 13–14). Health is social, and societies are defined by their power dynamics.

Power relationships take on special importance for population health science for two additional reasons. First, the field is still in its formative stage (Keyes and Galea 2016a), which means that it needs to settle on answers to many questions, including what healthcare's role is in the intersectoral project of population health science (see discussion in Chapter 6) and what epidemiology's role is in the interdisciplinary field (Labonté 1995; Evans and Stoddart 1990). Second, population health science is built around the notion that promoting population health requires a reworking of which parties contribute to the effort and how (Nash et al. 2016: xviii). Whether or not readers agree with Longino, that diffusion of power is a suitable principle in all scientific research, I want to stress that redistributing power is a central concern for population health science.

I will argue in this final chapter that humility is key to population health science's success. Humility is needed in three areas: an overarching epistemic humility recognizing that no single person or perspective can have a full understanding of population health; intersectoral humility recognizing that no sector of society (government, healthcare, etc.) is elevated above the others; and a disciplinary humility recognizing that no contributing discipline in interdisciplinary population health science is elevated above the others. After arguing for these points, drawing on previous chapters' arguments, I follow with a section discussing how the preceding sections relate to population health science education and conclude the book with some recommendations for future work in philosophy of population health.

Embracing epistemic humility

A key lesson of Part 1 of this book is the need for every actor involved in population health science to adopt a humble acceptance that population health knowledge and expertise are spread piecemeal across many different knowers. In this vein, Anita Ho defines the concept "epistemic humility" as rooted in:

> professionals' acknowledgment of the boundary of their expert domain as well as their fallibility. It means a commitment to make realistic assessment of what one knows and does not know, and to restrict one's confidence and claims to knowledge only to what one actually knows about his/her specialized domain.
>
> (Ho 2011: 117)

> Epistemic humility in health professionals is characterized by a commitment to mutual "collaboration and trust" with those they serve.
>
> (Ho 2011: 115)

In contrast to the ideal of epistemic humility, the powerful healthcare-centered biomedical model of health is an inescapably hierarchical model of health knowledge and expertise. Advocates of this model can certainly be respectful in their interactions with all manner of health experts. But, at the end of the day the model is committed to certain beliefs about what health is (matters of objective fact about biological/chemical/physical components of human bodies) and how it should be investigated and intervened upon (via experimental methods, preferably using advanced technology and laboratory techniques, seeking to reduce complex wholes to the sums of their parts) (Krieger 2011: 130). In such a model, patients are at best a means of transmitting hard-to-detect knowledge about their own bodies (e.g., their level of pain), rather than possessors of an irreplaceable set of knowledge and judgments (e.g., the causal factors for, and current status of, their spiritual well-being).[1] Much rides on the who-where-when-why-how of trust in other's knowledge. This issue comes to head in the philosophical literature disputing how much to trust people's testimony about their own health.

Epistemic humility is not the same thing as epistemic skepticism—it is not simply an assertion that we are all limited knowers. Epistemic humility is about curbing hubris and replacing egotism and pride with a "realistic" (Ho 2011: 117), and unsparing, evaluation of the knowledge-related weaknesses of individuals and groups whose knowledge assertions are given excessive deference. The important second half of epistemic humility is applying the same unassuming scrutiny to the knowledge of individuals and groups whose knowledge assertions have been undervalued. One key tension at stake is the balance of health knowledge authority between a person's assessment of their own well-being vs. the assessments made by external medical science authorities.

Sen describes the tension in the balance between internal vs. external perspectives on health—the trade-offs between assessing health based on the reflexive perceptions of people experiencing their health (e.g., survey-reported well-being) or through external sets of health statistics (e.g., infant mortality rates) (Sen 2004). He insists that both are valuable components of a full understanding of health. By contrast, Hausman thinks it essential to constrain both the scope of what can qualify as human flourishing and also which aspects of one's own flourishing a person is qualified to assess.

> "flourishing" consists in the dynamic coherent integration of objective goods into an identity. Well-being is flourishing. Subjective experience is one indicator of whether someone is flourishing.
>
> (Hausman 2015: 141)

Hausman's representation of flourishing/well-being gives an important place to individual identity, but doubts people's access to, or understanding of, their own well-being.

> To the extent that people are evaluatively competent—which is to say, to the extent that their preferences manifest a coherent identity that is rich in objective goods—(and also rational, self-interested, and well-informed), their preferences are good evidence concerning their well-being.
>
> (Hausman 2015: 141)

In other words, Hausman only recognizes individual humans as competent judges of their own health to the extent that they manifest patently non-human idealizations (perfect rationality, unwavering self-interest, and being totally factually informed).

It is worth giving some closer attention to Hausman's claim that self-knowledge of one's own health is contingent on being "rational, self-interested, and well-informed" (Hausman 2015: 141), since it is a concise description of a common, but flawed, position that serves to inappropriately valorize dispassionate rationality. It ends up creating an epistemic standard of self-knowledge that is only achievable by a member of the mythical species *Homo economicus*, *Homo sapiens*' hyper-rational relative, whose only known habitat is introductory economics textbooks. Ironically, Siconolfi et al. have collected and analyzed interviews with young gay and bisexual men, poignantly illustrating that the "archetype of *homo economicus*, the autonomous entrepreneur acting purely in rational, self-interested ways" is both a poor representation of how the men in their sample actually behave, and that when the men nevertheless *endorse* such an ideal, the net effect is toxic to population health—it leads the men to accept and perpetuate social stigma and marginalization against fellow sexual minorities (Siconolfi et al. 2015: 564). Whether or not one wears a condom during sex depends on a plethora of interacting factors, including not just cost–benefit analyses but also one's resources (not least of all, money) and the subjectivity one has built up during a complete life course of social experiences. In other words, *Homo sapiens'* sexual habits do not much resemble those of *Homo economicus*, but some *Homo sapiens* insist on idealizing *Homo economicus* anyway. The net effect is a contrived social blindness to the ways that seemingly autonomous self-serving choices are contingent on variable and inequitable social conditions, and on the subjective standpoints of the people in those various conditions.

Hausman's notion of what constitutes an ideal "evaluatively competent" individual fails to even work as an ideal. Those who see only their own interests and countenance only rationalist thought are evaluatively *incompetent* judges of the epistemically crucial subjectivities and social contingencies of health and health knowledge. By contrast, population health science and the participatory methods therein are predicated on an empirically founded trust that real people are capable of self-knowledge, and that *the value of their self-knowledge is due to their inextricable embedding in dynamic social lives*, not in spite of that embedding. I know my social well-being deeply, and better than anyone else, because that well-being is the result of my everyday life. This issue overlaps with decades of work done under the ethical framework of "Ethics of Care," which rejects "seeing the person as rational, autonomous agent, or a self-interested individual" and instead pleads for attention to the empirical fact and ethical necessity of attending to humans' relationships with each other—"relations that are often laden with emotion and involuntary" (Held 2006: 13).

I take the time to discuss Hausman's highly restricted trust in the epistemic competence of people to know their own health contrasts here because it differs markedly from the philosophical commitments built into population health. He offers an argument for epistemic skepticism (grounds for doubting people's epistemic abilities as knowers of their own health), while I see population health science as better served by an epistemic humility that recognizes that others can know their domains even if they have radically different experiences and knowledge resources.

> Co-production of health implies co-production of knowledge. If governance for health is to be effective, it must be participatory and include, but transcend, expert opinion. People's experience and people's perceptions are beginning to count in new ways.
>
> (Kickbusch and Gleicher 2012: 14)

Population health thinking is an outgrowth of the aforementioned social and holistic understanding of health. As articulated by Labonté et al., the proper "epistemological basis for population health research" is a worldview that rejects the assumption that population health researchers can encounter an ailing population and—as wise objective outsiders—solve its problems using some universal tools of science. They offer an alternative view:

This participatory epistemology assumes that understanding can only be achieved through deliberate dialogue and reflection, recognizes the validity of experiential knowing and presumes the capacity of people to learn about and understand their worlds.

(Labonté et al. 2005: 10–11)

A population's lay members have expertise about that population's health. Full stop.

Disability studies scholars including Edwards and Amundson have made similar points about the ethical folly and epistemic hubris of disputing disabled people's testimony when they report having high levels of well-being (Edwards 2013; Amundson 2005). For example, Buchman et al. explain that epistemic humility is the proper beginning stance to take when addressing patient testimony about the nature and severity of their chronic pain (Buchman et al. 2017). Of course, individuals undergoing, and providing testimony about, an experience are not the only experts relevant to that experience. Physicians have relevant knowledge too, such as prognoses of how pain patterns are likely to change over time. The point here is that, if health arises through the nuanced interactions between individuals and social structures, then it would be foolish to disregard the expertise of those who spend their lives navigating those social structures. Along similar lines, Galarneau pointedly criticizes the dominant health equity literature, including (Powers and Faden 2006; Daniels 2008; Ruger 2010), for reinforcing the marginalization of some community members, in part by creating philosophical theories in which "communities are *not* cast as heterogeneous and dynamic entities composed of morally authoritative community members who participate in just health care decision making" (Galarneau 2016: 37).

An epistemically humble approach to population health science goes hand in hand with a respect for the power of social contingency. Epistemic hubris appears in scientific reasoning when one presumes that a correct scientific claim is inevitable in the sense that "any other properly-resourced and rigorously-conducted investigation of the same subject matter" would reach the same conclusion (Kidd 2016: 13). It is hubris to believe that population health science is the relentless process of converging on objective universal truths; alternatively, population health science with a proper degree of epistemic humility recognizes that attempts to understand and promote health in the enormously diverse populations of the world must be well prepared to find that the best population health science practices (e.g., community-based participatory research) may end up looking quite different in varying locales. Moreover, we ought not attempt to force methods to convergence on a single set of universal best practices.

Much about the health of populations defies universal generalization. Population health science's knowledge is, to a large extent, local.

We are, by definition, concerned with the determination of the health of populations—a determination that is ineluctably linked to context. If we are to understand what matters most, we must understand how a particular factor matters within the broader context in which it appears.

(Galea 2018: 171)

Nancy McHugh has shown this in her book, *The Limits of Knowledge*—the book is structured as a series of case studies which do not lend themselves well to tidy generalizations, though, one general lesson McHugh draws is that Krieger's ecosocial model of health is the most promising model for rigorously and responsibly approaching public health knowledge (McHugh 2015). Krieger's work under the ecosocial model, as described repeatedly in the preceding chapters, is one particularly rigorous and complete manifestation of population health science theory (Krieger 2011). It is a generalization that works *because* it respects local contingency.

The problem of generalizability of knowledge touches upon many areas of population health science. In articulating her philosophical approach on the tension between local knowledge, McHugh criticizes the rigidity of evidence-based medicine. As I say in Chapter 6, evidence-based medicine has so far offered too little to population health, but I am more sanguine than McHugh about the future prospects of synchronizing evidence-based medicine with equitable health promotion efforts, including serving the marginalized minority populations that McHugh rightly worries about being underserved (McHugh 2015: 66–71). As described in Chapter 6's case study on the health of migrants, Bhopal makes clear that some of the problem could be rectified with devoting additional resources to equity in evidence-based medicine (Bhopal 2014: 217). As Kohatsu et al. described over a decade ago, the most promising way to carry out more equitable evidence-based public health research is to reshape the research process to more explicitly account for local preferences, with community-based participatory research being "one promising framework" for doing this (Kohatsu et al. 2004). More recently, the GRADE guidelines used in assessing the quality of evidence in evidence-based medicine have been updated to more explicitly incorporate assessment of health equity, since the overall quality of a piece of evidence for a given purpose is contingent on how relevant that data is to the experiences and needs of the populations that are now underserved (Welch et al. 2017). It is possible to make evidence-based medicine more sensitive to the diverse experiences and needs distributed within and between populations. Making general inferences, while also respecting the power of local contingency, is an enduring challenge, not a reason to give up in despair. In short, population health science knowledge is very much contingent, local, social, and multifaceted. No one has a firm grasp on the full scope of knowledge about a given population health case. For example, the Chapter 7 case study featuring the UK Prevention of Diabetes of South Asians (PODOSA) program shows how it was essential for researchers to work in a spirit of epistemic humility with the populations they strive to serve—building the sort of "bidirectional collaboration and trust" advocated by Ho (Ho 2011: 115; Bhopal et al. 2014; Morrison et al. 2014).

Epistemic humility can quite reasonably inspire a sense of dread for those who wish to efficiently use the limited resources of population health science to generate universal principles that can be applied to any given case. As discussed in Chapter 2, formulating effective methods of community-based participatory research remains a highly active enterprise, and one that is fraught with inevitable frustrations (Freudenberg and Tsui 2014). If complex social dynamics are powerful causal factors for health outcomes, and if members of a population are experts in the social dynamics of their own population, then those members of the population have important expertise in the causation of their population's health. Embracing epistemic humility also advances the population health science goal of addressing health's upstream social causes. Chapter 3 shows why an adequate conceptualization and implementation of health and disease concepts requires genuine and humble engagement with the communities that will ultimately have those concepts applied to them, as illustrated in the case of Aboriginal Australians' health. Chapters 4 and 5 argue for the need to address the powerful underlying causes of disease embedded in social dynamics, such as racism and other "fundamental causes" of health (Phelan and Link 2015). Population health science practitioners must choose where they will stand in the zone between epistemic hubris and epistemic humility; I urge them to prefer the epistemic humility side.

Sectoral humility: non-hierarchical intersectorality

"Population health and equity depend upon collaborative, intersectoral action" (Rudolph et al. 2013: 17). Health—*a life course trajectory of complete well-being in social context* (as defined in Chapter 3)—is woven through every corner of social life. Well-being's causes and effects are everywhere. Accordingly, no single sector of society can claim ultimate ownership over health matters. Take diet, an important piece of the larger whole of health. No matter how one divides up the sectors of society, virtually every sector of society has some rightful claim on diet as being within their domain: agriculture, transportation, the food service industry, religions, healthcare, local community organizations, government, etc. In light of the diffuse and socially embedded nature of health as an entity and object of intervention (Chapters 3 and 4), health's upstream social causes and innumerable effects (Chapter 5) and the nature of health equity and governance as bound up in all efforts to study and intervene upon health (Chapter 7), I propose the following: all sectors of society must embrace humility if we are to be effective collaborators in promoting health.

No sector of society sits at the top of the hierarchy of population health collaborators. Doctors, clerics, and politicians may be some of the most common perpetrators of health hubris in recent history, but it is no less problematic for community activist leaders, pharmaceutical CEOs or any other representative of a sector of society to seek to elevate that sector above all others. In the face of the staggering immensity of health as a phenomenon, and health promotion as an objective, the proper response for each sector is to embrace humility. Good population health not only takes all sectors of society working together, but there is no rightful "first among equals" in population health intersectorality.

Chapter 6 discusses the tension of population health efforts that build intersectorality outward from the healthcare sector vs. population health efforts that seek to decenter healthcare entirely when building up efforts to promote health intersectorally. The deep challenge is moving from a model of health promotion dominated by healthcare (which varies by location in how much it lines up with private industry—my country, the US, is an extreme example of for-profit healthcare dominance) to an intersectoral model. The consequences of this dominance are frustratingly illustrated in the dialogue between Kindig and Isham and respondents in a special issue of *Frontiers of Health Services Management*. Kindig (the population health leader featured often in this book) and Isham had contributed a featured article describing how healthcare business leaders could integrate their companies' missions to make them productive parts of a larger intersectoral effort to promote population health (Kindig and Isham 2014a). After a series of commentaries all discussing how to make healthcare improvements, the seemingly exasperated authors replied, "our succinct, summary response would be '… but it's not primarily about medical care'" (Kindig and Isham 2014b: 56). Such is the challenge of coaxing individual sectors of society to work within an intersectoral model in which no one sector rules the others. Kindig and Isham's struggle to convey this to the healthcare sector in many ways mirrors Goldberg's struggle to convince Rothstein that government mandates need not be the drivers of public health or population health efforts (Goldberg 2009; Rothstein 2009).

The politics of intersectorality are difficult to manage at best. Chapter 6's discussion of balancing methodological trade-offs in population health shows the perils of erring too far on the side of either ideological purity (at the expense of making population health progress alongside partially likeminded partners) or on the side of short-term pragmatism (achieving some concrete goals through partnering with somewhat likeminded partners but at the expense of hampering long-term goals, such as the goal of moving from a healthcare sector-dominated model to a more intersectoral model of health promotion). It appears that the creditable (and linked) projects of the Social Medicine discipline and the People's Health Movement have both sacrificed much by erring on the side of ideological restrictiveness in their strategies. Population health stands to succeed where those other efforts have proven themselves to be self-limiting. Nash et al.'s textbook of population health is perhaps the most cogent and confident articulation of what it means to hold onto social justice commitments in population health (inclusivity, care for the economically disadvantaged, concern about the social repercussions of economic inequality, etc.) while still featuring chapters such as "Making The Case For Population Health Management: The Business Value Of A Healthy Workforce" (Nash et al. 2016).

The move from older models of public health to a humbly intersectoral population health science requires overt and transparent dialogue about intersectorality as a political reform. Rose was prescient and bold when he told the public health science community that it needed to choose between a "radical" and transformative scientific agenda or a piecemeal and narrow one (Rose 1985, 1992). He died not long after outlining this, so he never saw that this radical agenda—investigating the causes of population-level health disparities and seeking to reshape society accordingly—eventually coalesced into the field of population health science (Keyes and Galea 2016a; Nash et al. 2016). The alternative to Rose's population health endeavor is the de facto conservatism of saying that public health must stay constrained to a narrow set of actions by government and healthcare sectors (Epstein 2003; Rothstein 2009). The sectoral conservatism of propping up the "old public health" is especially dangerous if its advocates fail to acknowledge the associated political conservatism of defending laissez-faire capitalism and individualism, while opposing collective social and economic reforms (Gostin and Bloche 2003). Ironically though, the (sometimes romanticized) narrow model of twentieth-century "old public health" never consistently exemplified those ethical and political principles anyway, if one examines the history critically and unromantically (Novak 2003). The narrow model of public health of narrow exercise of government authority gleefully carried out flagrant abuses of power, such as mandatory eugenic sterilizations and racist campaigns to destroy the housing of stigmatized immigrants, and otherwise use fully authorized government powers to intimidate and attack socially marginalized people (Novak 2003). As Rose surmised (Rose 1985, 1992), radical political reforms now look like the only viable means to effectively promoting populations' health.

Public health's nineteenth-century founders seem to have had a keener sense of the need to pursue activism across sectors of society than most of the twentieth-century scholars who followed them (Freudenberg and Tsui 2014; Krieger and Birn 1998; Krieger 2011; Ståhl et al. 2006). Population health science influence in the twenty-first century has shifted the dominant ideology. Chapter 4 shows that broad models of public/population health are now thoroughly mainstream. Models such as Health in all Policies have become increasingly appealing as evidence of health's social causation has accumulated (World Health Organization 2015).

A humble and collaborative spirit of intersectorality is looking like the way forward in light of the inescapably political work that needs to be done. Singh's book, *Dying and Living in the Neighborhood* turns attention to neighborhoods in making the case for intersectoral collaboration, offering neighborhood-level programs as a bottom-up alternative to failed top-down health policies (Singh 2016). Popko (a Catholic nun) uses population health science theory to elaborate on the need for intersectoral responses to health inequities, articulating how Catholics in the religious sector and in the healthcare sector have roles to play (Popko 2015). The illustrative examples go on. There is much political reform work that must be done, humbly and together.

Disciplinary humility: non-hierarchical interdisciplinarity

Population health science is an interdisciplinary field of study and framework for thinking about health. It remains unresolved whether population health science will or should become a totally distinct cohesive interdiscipline, in the sense that biochemistry is its own (inter)discipline and not just the science done in the area of overlap between biology and chemistry (Klein 1990: 43). This is not to say that the formation of an interdiscipline is progress per se; Klein makes a good case that building an interdiscipline is not inherently superior to other forms of interdisciplinarity (Klein 1990: 43). Population health science certainly *could* become an interdiscipline. It has textbooks (e.g., Nash et al. 2016) and journals (e.g., *Population Health Management* and *Social Science & Medicine— Population Health*); at the institutional level, there are academic units such as the Jefferson University College of Population Health and the Population Health PhD offered at the University of Ottawa. Meanwhile, new academic *centers* for population health sciences are opening their doors (Lee 2016; Scheibal 2015), which seems quite natural since centers are typically trans-departmental and transdisciplinary by design. But centers face a particular set of perils owing to limited funding, hiring power, and other administrative obstacles (Glied et al. 2007). No one model of population health science interdisciplinarity is clearly the right one. Population health science has always been interdisciplinary and I defer to pluralism on the question of whether population health science ought to become an interdiscipline (housed in colleges/departments) or a field pursued in the liminal space between other disciplines; for the time being, let there be both! I see this as in keeping with Diez Roux's pragmatic shrug at the question of whether population health science is a different thing than a suitably reformed public health science—"the more synonyms we have, the better" (Diez Roux 2016: 620).

Since its earliest days, population health science has struggled to build a field that is suitably inclusive of the many disciplines it needs as contributors. In the early days of the field, Labonté criticized Evans and Stoddart's stance on the disciplinary primacy of epidemiology (Labonté 1995; Evans and Stoddart 1990). Epidemiology has long enjoyed pride of place in the interdisciplinary field of public health science; it "is commonly referred to as the foundation of public health" (Merrill 2017: 2). That elevated position is inappropriate in population health science. In the population health science milestone Leeds Declaration, of the ten items in the declaration, four are pleas for pluralistic interdisciplinarity. The Declaration calls for a "plurality of methods," and an "openness to the contribution of a variety of disciplines," rejecting the disparagement of "qualitative data" and condemning assertions that such methods are "soft" while "quantitative" sciences are "hard" (The Lancet Editors 1994). Even more distressingly, epidemiology's elevated disciplinary position in public health science seems to be an extension of the field's lingering ivory tower habits. Dowdy and Pai surmise that epidemiologists have become more and more concerned with objectivity and methods for attributing causality, effectively neglecting the crucial matters of clinical translation, community engagement, policymaking support, and education (Dowdy and Pai 2012). I support their call for epidemiologists to instead take up the professional role of "accountable health advocate," insofar as this means they must be just one of several types of advocate working toward the common goal of population health improvement.

Integrating the different contributions of different disciplines in an interdisciplinary effort faces deep-seated philosophical obstacles, yet there is ample reason to be optimistic that the obstacles can be overcome. Brister helpfully divides up the types of epistemic disagreements that obstruct interdisciplinary collaborations: "1. facts, 2. evidentiary standards or 'rigor,' 3. causes, and 4. research goals" (Brister 2016: 84). Since the interdisciplinary challenges are bone deep, so to speak, solutions will require ongoing participatory dialogue among the many parties. Solutions will require addressing matters such as whether we have sufficient data to justify population health proposals to mandate minimum pricing for a unit of alcohol, and if not then what would constitute sufficient evidence? On this sort of question, Marmot's UN Commission points the way forward by embracing a pragmatic pluralism about population health evidence.

> The Commission took a broader view of what constituted evidence … In this report the reader will find evidence that comes from observational studies (including natural experiments and cross-country studies), case studies, and field visits, from expert and lay knowledge, and from community intervention trials where available.
>
> (Commission on Social Determinants of Health 2008: 42)

No single discipline or method can claim primacy in population health's interdisciplinary efforts, a necessary pluralism that is reinforced by the fact that practical limitations will force researchers to venture farther from their comfort zones when gathering relevant evidence.

Longino explains that diffusion of power is a feminist goal, for both epistemic reasons and ethical ones (Longino 1995). She endorses several scientific power diffusion efforts, including proposals to recognize midwifery as applied science and other medical practices that empower women as the controllers of their own bodies—these efforts have made considerable progress (McClimans 2015; Every Woman Every Child 2015). A humble interdisciplinary approach to population health science serves to radically advance these same sorts of power diffusion goals by redistributing the underlying power dynamics of scientific disciplines and their associated professions.

Health science experts of many kinds are set to gain from the decentralization of disciplinary power in population health science, while physicians correspondingly lose their elevated stature in individual-level health science and epidemiologists lose their elevated stature in individual-level health science. Nurses are set to play expanded roles in health promotion, partly since nurses occupy a liminal professional space between traditional biomedical institutions (especially hospitals) and the populations being served (MacDonald et al. 2013; Bekemeier 2008). And, it is worth noting that nursing is a traditionally female occupation— further evidence that Longino was right to see power diffusion as a feminist "theoretical virtue" and a means of empowering women (Longino 1995). But other marginalized health professions gain as well. Dental professionals of all kinds have new work to do once we recognize "the importance of a life-course approach and ... the wider determinants of health," allowing us to reanalyze and reconfigure interventions to address the oral health inequities that arise from which detrimental oral health exposures a population's members experience, and when, over the life course (Batchelor 2012: 12). Torres et al. show that many wealthy countries with sophisticated centralized healthcare systems have woefully failed to recognize the huge range of essential roles played by a diverse set of frontline "community health workers" (Torres et al. 2014). These community health workers form the very frontline of many population health functions, since they are (by definition) members of a relevant community (e.g., an immigrant) who do paid or unpaid population health promotion tasks such as helping fellow community members to access health resources, or serving as "multicultural health brokers" (e.g., a de facto mediator of information flow between an ethnic minority immigrant community and the policymakers) (Torres et al. 2014). This diffusion of power meshes with the notion of health as social, discussed in Chapter 2. As the Ottawa Charter puts it, "health is created and lived by people within the settings of their everyday life; where they learn, work, play and love" (World Health Organization 1986). Accordingly, population health science ought to continue redistributing authority away from the few highly credentialed health experts (the relatively small ranks of epidemiologists and physicians) and redistributing that authority to the many forms of knowledge/ expertise crucial to understanding and intervening in the messy social realities of health. Such a project of redistributing disciplinary authority quickly raises the question of what such a shifting power redistribution means for how health experts are educated.

Population health science education for health professionals

Interdisciplinarity and cross-sectoral collaboration is the best solution to Rothstein's objection that public health experts lack training in how to address fundamental societal causes of populations' health problems (Rothstein 2002). Individual public health practitioners may typically lack advanced training in working individually or collaboratively on policy matters, but that indeed helped motivate the creation of population health science in the first place. The solution to inadequate education isn't giving up; the solution is better education! Among many other efforts, faculty from the Jefferson University College of Population Health Science have made strides toward filling the educational gap by creating a college and a textbook (Nash et al. 2011, 2016). Along similar lines, Duke University has offered a roadmap of the population health learning goals needed for health professionals to be competent in the principles of population health

(Kaprielian et al. 2013). Many public health professionals are not adequately prepared for, or integrated in, policymaking. Population health science offers the daunting but achievable solution: change how we do health science training. As mentioned in Chapter 1, the 2016 accrediting standards for US public health higher education programs make frequent reference to "population health" (a change from the 2011 standards, which did not), including the requirement that Master's-level and Doctoral-level education must, "substantively address scientific and analytic approaches to discovery and translation of public health knowledge in the context of a population health framework" (Council on Education for Public Health 2016: 29). The challenge ahead is complex in many ways, including philosophically.

A radical change in health education is necessitated by the theoretical and disciplinary shifts offered by population health science. May, a leading scholar of clinical bioethics, declares with two population health colleagues in the journal *Population Health Management*:

> [Population health management] dissolves the traditional distinction of clinical medicine and public health … PHM represents a new paradigm for understanding the fiduciary duties within the physician and patient relationship.
>
> (May et al. 2017: 168–169)

They argue that one the greatest virtues of the "paradigm" is its successful bridging of individual health and population health, leading it to "embrace the symbiotic relationship between these individual and population realms traditionally perceived to compete and/or balance against each other" (May et al. 2017: 169). Population health has successfully spread the reach of public health thinking downward, into the realm of individual clinical practice. Fortunately, a humble intersectoral and interdisciplinary response has been offered for the education of physicians and other health practitioners working in individual clinical care: the adoption of "structural competence" (Reich et al. 2016).

Reich, Hansen, and Link—the latter a co-creator of Fundamental Cause Theory, featured in Chapter 5—argue in a 2016 *Bioethical Inquiry* article that the theory should shape not only population-level policy but also individual clinical care and education of clinicians (Reich et al. 2016). Individualistic thinking in health may benefit single patients or improve median health outcomes, but could end up actually adding to inequitable distributions of health burdens (Reich et al. 2016).

> A fundamental cause perspective suggests that clinicians' focus on individual-level interventions likely exacerbates health inequalities even as it may improve health in the aggregate. Thus, structural competency is not only necessary in order for clinicians to properly address their patients' needs but also ethically significant in that it might result in greater health equity.
>
> (Reich et al. 2016: 191)

Until physicians have such structural competencies, they are not adequately trained for the business of caring for patients. After all, how could a physician be expected to do an adequate job if they were unaware that health's causes start far upstream from, and far outside the traditional purview of, the clinic?

Incorporating structural competence, and an interest in structural interventions, expands the epistemic purview of clinicians, even as it responds to their limited power. They have more to understand and to do than typically recognized, because their traditional activities are simply not powerful enough. Clinicians must only search the patient's body and behaviors for causes of disease, but also the much wider social contexts: minimum wage laws, public transit access, restrictions on social welfare access, etc. Reich et al. see no alternative to demanding that physicians add this to their already daunting list of basic competencies and I agree (Reich et al. 2016). Individual physicians may lack the power to change the lack of public transportation in a city, but Reich et al. help to show why they have a professional duty to try.

Rather than seeing structural competency as an effort to pursue in isolation, it is just one important prong of a multi-pronged strategy. The "Population Health Across All Professions" report by the Association of Schools and Programs of Public Health stresses that population health education must simultaneously target curricula in all disciplines whose professionals wittingly or unwittingly play important roles in population health causation: "e.g., law, business, architecture, urban planning, teaching and engineering" (Association of Schools and Programs of Public Health 2015: 3). To repeat, humble intersectoral and interdisciplinary collaboration are essential. Such efforts must include all health professionals, and also extend beyond them too. Laypeople's education needs reform as well.

Population health science education for all

"Population health" and "population health science" are terms understood by few outside the health professions, and even inside the health professions, the process of defining and communicating the concepts has been slow (MHA@GW Staff 2015; Keyes and Galea 2016b). Population health experts' communication with the lay public has been unsuccessful, and constitutes the most glaring failure of population health science. There are notable attempts to address this, such as Galea's active efforts to share population health science thinking via his highly accessible public blog and the published volume based on it (Galea 2018). Such efforts acknowledged, the population health framework is effectively an open secret, debated in health experts' writings to each other, with very little outreach done to communicate the framework to lay publics.

It will not be an easy or safe process. Public health education efforts can easily go awry. Briggs and Hallin show how contemporary media coverage produces new understandings of health, not just the filtering and distribution of ideas produced by biomedical experts (Briggs and Hallin 2016). Among those ways is the de facto growth of a murky zone of overlap between biomedicine and mass media, reflecting media interest in health stories and biomedical institutions' interests in media assistance in communicating with publics (Briggs and Hallin 2016). I take this as a reason to embrace the de facto reality and include media as one of the sectors invited to the table during population health deliberations. This is only one of many steps needed for population health practitioners to communicate their overarching goals and methods to lay publics.

I suspect that some of the reason for population health science's failure to earn widespread recognition is due to the science's inherent local contingency, as discussed in the first half of this chapter. Local population health efforts, if pursued in properly participatory fashion, need to expend much effort in communicating what that population health intervention is, what motivates it, and how it aims to achieve its population health goals. In individual cases such as the model of population health promotion that Western Australia developed for its Aboriginal population, expounded in the Chapter 3 case study, there was necessarily a large component of stakeholder education (Government of Western Australia Department of Health 2015). There is no corresponding routine process or responsible party for communicating about population health science *as a whole* to the public as a whole.

The Triple Aim framework for healthcare-centered population health proposes a solution, designating a certain entity to serve as the "integrator" charged with seeing the big picture and working toward overcoming disciplinary and institutional gaps, including taking chief responsibility for facilitating education and communication efforts (Berwick et al. 2008). I am skeptical of this education mechanism. In addition to the worries I articulate in Chapter 6 about the healthcare sector perhaps having disproportionate power in the Triple Aim framework, I am also concerned about the way that the integrator role combines communication and education tasks with responsibility for resource allocation and other managerial roles. Concentrating governance power into a single entity is a risky move at best. It conflicts with the recommendation that intersectoral collaboration be pursued *without* a hierarchy. Several existing de facto integrators are cited in support of the Triple Aim proposal to appoint more such integrators. Of the cited examples, some have far better claims to democratic governance legitimacy (the National Health Service in the UK) than others (health maintenance organizations—a type of health insurance provider—in the US) (Berwick et al. 2008).

Even if an integrator can successfully incorporate the insights of the many sectors and disciplines, it is essential that any overarching governing entity have the right to govern and the ability to do so in a manner that properly manifests the humble and collaborative spirit needed for the philosophically sound application of population health science. The Institute of Medicine's 2016 report on educating health professionals about social determinants of health includes a call to "put the community in charge of taking actions to assess and improve population health and the wellbeing of the community" (Committee on Educating Health Professionals to Address the Social Determinants of Health 2016: 53). A community can be "in charge" via a collective decision to cede managerial functions to a given entity, but under a population health science framework, communities are the proper beneficiaries of empowerment efforts. Even government efforts must (humbly) take into account that governmental policies are also best developed via intersectoral collaboration (Potvin and Jones 2011; World Health Organization 1986). Again, I advocate for non-hierarchical intersectoral collaboration.

In the meantime, population health science remains a hazy or unknown entity for most. This failure of communication is all the more unacceptable because it is inconsistent with population health science theory. Transparency and open lines of communication between all parties involved in population health issues are vital components of the science. There is a poignant ethical irony in the fact that population health, built on a philosophical foundation of participatory and collaborative commitments, pursues these commitments while the vast majority of the people they serve remain unaware of what those commitments are, why they are embraced, and why they matter. It is an unacceptable status quo.

Lest this sound like another high-minded and empty-headed call for solving complex problems via the failed "deficit model" of science education ("the public lacks knowledge—deliver it to them and all will work out") I stress that sharing the vision of population health science must serve to initiate ongoing dialogues, not a set of patronizing one-way monologues. Multidirectional information sharing is ethically and epistemically essential (Soranno et al. 2015). More broadly, public education is not a panacea. As briefly covered in Chapter 6, education interventions can be some of the most problematic because education efforts are most effective among those who have already benefitted from solid educations, meaning that education efforts are prone to exacerbating the marginalization and exclusion of those who most need to be included (Phelan et al. 2010; Frohlich and Potvin 2008). Taking population health science out of the shadows of Academia is a starting point, not an ending point.

Philosophy of population health from a position of service

Population health has many known and unknown challenges ahead, and this final chapter of the book has argued that population health ought to embrace humility and a spirit of collaboration as it confronts those challenges. As individual knowers, all who take an interest in population health would be wise to embrace epistemic humility—to recognize their limited abilities to understand the dizzying complexity of population health. A thoroughly non-hierarchical and humble ethic of intersectoral collaboration is needed to escape the inadequate narrow and biomedicine-dominated model of health as belonging to government and healthcare. Similarly, population health science's internal disciplinary dynamics are best served by a thoroughly non-hierarchical and humble ethic of interdisciplinary collaboration. No discipline ought to dominate population health science, whether or not one envisions population health science as a discrete (inter)discipline of its own. The long-overdue efforts to educate health professionals and the lay public must be similarly careful to manifest spirits of humility and collaboration.

I hope that this book as a whole has exemplified the collaborative humility that I endorse in this chapter. The first chapter states this is a book on philosophy of population health as philosophy *for* population health—"philosophy from the position of service" (Dotson 2015). This is a service that must be done collaboratively. Philosophy of population health must be "broad and inclusive" for the same sorts of reasons that Keyes and Galea say population health science should be such:

> First, scholars from different disciplines are coming together as population health scientists, bringing with them different perspectives and approaches. Second, the challenges that population health science tackles of necessity require engagement with a breadth of concepts and methods to approach complex, solution-resistant problems.
>
> (Keyes and Galea 2016b: 633)

"A breadth of concepts and methods" are necessary to address the philosophical aspects of a field that is itself composed of "a breadth of concepts and methods."

I hope that this book's philosophical analysis will be followed by other focused works on philosophy of population health. Whatever my colleagues think about what population health is, could be, or should be, I at least hope that that this book has made the case for giving more focused attention to population health and population health science. Assuming that this book does draw more attention to the philosophical aspects of population health, I urge the philosophers and non-philosophers who take interest in those matters to not dismiss the philosophical insights of non-philosophers. Population health science is unusually overt in its philosophical content, a theme I hope has been conveyed throughout this book. Population health science has been reevaluating—and taking important philosophical stances on—what population health is, what causes population health, who should research and intervene in population health and how, what obstacles face ethical population health promotion and what ethical population health is in the first place. I see overwhelming reasons to urge population health science to continue in its current direction. Population health scholars have done an admirable job of addressing a wide variety of philosophical issues since the 1990s, and I hope this book aids in the efforts of understanding and addressing the many unresolved challenges now and in the future.

Note

1 Some deficits among biomedical model adherents are incidental to the model itself. For example, Solomon criticizes attempts to dichotomize narrative medicine as the caring, personal and humanistic alternative to the impersonal biomedical model—impersonal clinical encounters can have as much to do with a physician's mood as their philosophical commitments: Solomon (2015).

Works cited

Amundson, R. (2005) Disability, Ideology, and Quality of Life. In: Wasserman, D., Bickenbach, J. and Wachbroit, R. (eds) *Quality of Life and Human Difference. Genetic Testing, Health Care and Disability.* Cambridge: Cambridge University Press, 101–120.

Association of Schools and Programs of Public Health. (2015) Population Health across All Professions: Expert Panel Report. *Framing the Future.* Association of Schools and Programs of Public Health.

Batchelor, P. (2012) What do we mean by population health? *Community Dentistry and Oral Epidemiology* 40, 12–15.

Bekemeier, B. (2008) "Upstream" nursing practice and research. *Applied Nursing Research* 21, 50–52.

Berwick, D. M., Nolan, T. W. and Whittington, J. (2008) The Triple Aim: Care, health, and cost. *Health Affairs* 27, 759–769.

Bhopal, R. S. (2014) *Migration, Ethnicity, Race, and Health in Multicultural Societies.* Oxford: Oxford University Press.

Bhopal, R. S., Douglas, A., Wallia, S., et al. (2014) Effect of a lifestyle intervention on weight change in South Asian individuals in the UK at high risk of type 2 diabetes: A family-cluster randomised controlled trial. *The Lancet Diabetes & Endocrinology* 2, 218–227.

Briggs, C. L. and Hallin, D. C. (2016) *Making Health Public: How News Coverage Is Remaking Media, Medicine, and Contemporary Life.* Oxon: Routledge.

Brister, E. (2016) Disciplinary capture and epistemological obstacles to interdisciplinary research: Lessons from central African conservation disputes. *Studies in History and Philosophy of Biological and Biomedical Sciences* 56, 82–91.

Buchman, D. Z., Ho, A. and Goldberg, D. S. (2017) Investigating trust, expertise, and epistemic injustice in chronic pain. *Journal of Bioethical Inquiry* 14, 31–42.

Commission on Social Determinants of Health. (2008) Closing the Gap in a Generation: Health Equity Through Action on the Social Determinants of Health. Geneva: World Health Organization.

Committee on Educating Health Professionals to Address the Social Determinants of Health. (2016) A Framework for Educating Health Professionals to Address the Social Determinants of Health. Washington, DC: National Academies Press.

Council on Education for Public Health. (2016) Accreditation Criteria: Schools of Public Health & Public Health Programs. Silver Spring, MD: Council on Education for Public Health.

Daniels, N. (2008) *Just Health: Meeting Health Needs Fairly.* New York: Cambridge University Press.

Diez Roux, A. V. (2016) On the distinction—or lack of distinction—between population health and public health. *American Journal of Public Health* 106, 619–620.

Dotson, K. (2015) Philosophy from the Position of Service. In: Krishnamurthy, M. (ed.) *Philosopher.*

Dowdy, D. W. and Pai, M. (2012) Bridging the gap between knowledge and health: The epidemiologist as accountable health advocate ("AHA!"). *Epidemiology* 23, 914–918.

Edwards, C. (2013) The anomalous wellbeing of disabled people: A response. *Topoi* 32, 189–196.

Epstein, R. A. (2003) Let the shoemaker stick to his last: A defense of the "old" public health. *Perspectives in Biology and Medicine* 46, S138–S159.

Evans, R. G. and Stoddart, G. L. (1990) Producing health, consuming health care. *Social Science and Medicine* 31, 1347–1363.

Every Woman Every Child. (2015) The global strategy for women's, children's and adolescents' health. United Nations.

Freudenberg, N. and Tsui, E. (2014) Evidence, power, and policy change in community-based participatory research. *American Journal of Public Health* 104, 11–14.

Frohlich, K. L. and Potvin, L. (2008) Transcending the known in public health practice— the inequality paradox: The population approach and vulnerable populations. *American Journal of Public Health* 98, 216–221.

Galarneau, C. (2016) *Communities of Health Care Justice*. New Brunswick, NJ: Rutgers University Press.

Galea, S. (2018) *Healthier: Fifty Thoughts on the Foundations of Population Health*. New York: Oxford University Press.

Glied, S., Bakken, S., Formicola, A., et al. (2007) Institutional challenges of interdisciplinary research centers. *Journal of Research Administration* 38, 28–36.

Goldberg, D. S. (2009) In support of a broad model of public health: Disparities, social epidemiology and public health causation. *Public Health Ethics* 2, 70–83.

Gostin, L. O. and Bloche, M. G. (2003) The politics of public health: A response to Epstein. *Perspectives in Biology and Medicine* 46, S160–S175.

Government of Western Australia Department of Health. (2015) WA Aboriginal Health and Wellbeing Framework 2015–2030. http://ww2.health.wa.gov.au/Improving-WA-Health/About-Aboriginal-Health/WA-Aboriginal-Health-and-Wellbeing-Framework-2015-2030: Department of Health.

Hausman, D. M. (2015) *Valuing Health: Well-Being, Freedom and Suffering*. New York: Oxford University Press.

Held, V. (2006) *The Ethics of Care: Personal, Political, and Global*. New York: Oxford University Press.

Ho, A. (2011) Trusting experts and epistemic humility in disability. *International Journal of Feminist Approaches to Bioethics* 4, 102–123.

Kaprielian, V. S., Silberberg, M., McDonald, M. A., et al. (2013) Teaching population health: A competency map approach to education. *Academic Medicine* 88, 626–637.

Keyes, K. M. and Galea, S. (2016a) *Population Health Science*. New York: Oxford University Press.

Keyes, K. M. and Galea, S. (2016b) Setting the agenda for a new discipline: Population health science. *American Journal of Public Health* 106, 633–634.

Kickbusch, I. and Gleicher, D. (2012) *Governance for Health in the 21st Century*. Copenhagen: World Health Organization Regional Office for Europe.

Kidd, I. J. (2016) Inevitability, contingency, and epistemic humility. *Studies in History and Philosophy of Science* 55, 12–19.

Kindig, D. A. and Isham, G. (2014a) Population health improvement: A community health business model that engages partners in all sectors. *Frontiers of Health Services Management* 30, 3–20.

Kindig, D. A. and Isham, G. (2014b) Response from feature authors. *Frontiers of Health Services Management* 30, 56–57.

Klein, J. T. (1990) *Interdisciplinarity: History, Theory, and Practice*. Detroit, MI: Wayne State University Press.

Kohatsu, N. D., Robinson, J. G. and Torner, J. C. (2004) Evidence-based public health: An evolving concept. *American Journal of Preventive Medicine* 27, 417–421.

Krieger, N. (2011) *Epidemiology and the People's Health: Theory and Context*. New York: Oxford University Press.

Krieger, N. and Birn, A.-E. (1998) A vision of social justice as the foundation of public health: Commemorating 150 years of the spirit of 1848. *American Journal of Public Health* 88, 1603–1606.

Labonté, R. (1995) Population health and health promotion: What do they have to say to each other? *Canadian Journal of Public Health* 86, 165–168.

Labonté, R., Polanyi, M., Muhajarine, N., et al. (2005) Beyond the divides: Towards critical population health research. *Critical Public Health* 15, 5–17.

Lee, V. (2016) *Message from the Dean*. Available at: http://medicine.utah.edu/population-health-sciences/message-from-dean.php

Longino, H. E. (1995) Gender, politics, and the theoretical virtues. *Synthese* 104, 383–397.

MacDonald, S. E., Newburn-Cook, C. V., Allen, M. and Reutter, L. (2013) Embracing the population health framework in nursing research. *Nursing Inquiry* 20, 30–41.

May, T., Byonanebye, J. and Meurer, J. (2017) The ethics of population health management: Collapsing the traditional boundary between patient care and public health. *Population Health Management* 20, 167–169.

McClimans, L. (2015) Place of birth: Ethics and evidence. *Topoi*, 1–8.

McHugh, N. A. (2015) *The Limits of Knowledge: Generating Pragmatist Feminist Cases for Situated Knowing*. Albany, NY: SUNY Press.

Merrill, R. M. (2017) *Introduction to Epidemiology*. Burlington, MA: Jones and Bartlett Learning.

MHA@GW Staff. (2015) *What Is Population Health?* Available at: https://mha.gwu.edu/what-is-population-health/.

Morrison, Z., Douglas, A., Bhopal, R. and Sheikh, A. (2014) Understanding experiences of participating in a weight loss lifestyle intervention trial: A qualitative evaluation of South Asians at high risk of diabetes. *BMJ Open* 4, e004736.

Nash, D. B., Fabius, R. J., Skoufalos, A., et al. (2016) *Population Health: Creating a Culture of Wellness*. Second ed. Burlington, MA: Jones & Bartlett Learning.

Nash, D. B., Reifsnyder, J., Fabius, R. J., et al. (2011) *Population Health: Creating a Culture of Wellness*. Sudbury, MA: Jones & Bartlett Publishers.

Novak, W. J. (2003) Private wealth and public health: A critique of Richard Epstein's defense of the "old" public health. *Perspectives in Biology and Medicine* 46, S176–S198.

Phelan, J. C. and Link, B. G. (2015) Is racism a fundamental cause of inequalities in health? *Annual Review of Sociology* 41, 311–330.

Phelan, J. C., Link, B. G. and Tehranifar, P. (2010) Social conditions as fundamental causes of health inequalities: Theory, evidence, and policy implications. *Journal of Health and Social Behavior* 51, S28–S40.

Popko, K. (2015) The expanding advocacy agenda. *Health Progress*, 8–11.

Potvin, L. and Jones, C. M. (2011) Twenty-five years after the Ottawa Charter: The critical role of health promotion for public health. *Canadian Journal of Public Health* 102, 244–248.

Powers, M. and Faden, R. R. (2006) *Social Justice: The Moral Foundations of Public Health and Health Policy*. New York: Oxford University Press.

Reich, A. D., Hansen, H. B. and Link, B. G. (2016) Fundamental interventions: How clinicians can address the fundamental causes of disease. *Journal of Bioethical Inquiry* 13, 185–192.

Rose, G. (1985) Sick individuals and sick populations. *International Journal of Epidemiology* 14, 32–38.

Rose, G. (1992) *The Strategy of Preventive Medicine*. New York: Oxford University Press.

Rothstein, M. A. (2002) Rethinking the meaning of public health. *The Journal of Law, Medicine & Ethics* 30, 144–149.

Rothstein, M. A. (2009) The limits of public health: A response. *Public Health Ethics* 2, 84–88.

Rudolph, L., Caplan, J., Ben-Moshe, K. and Dillon, L. (2013) *Health in All Policies: A Guide for State and Local Governments*. Washington, DC: American Public Health Association and Public Health Institute.

Ruger, J. P. (2010) *Health and Social Justice*. Oxford: Oxford University Press.

Scheibal, S. (2015) *Dell Medical School Taps Medical Informatics Expert to Lead Population Health Department*. Available at: http://dellmedschool.utexas.edu/news/dell-medical-school-taps-medical-informatics-expert-to-lead-population-health-department.

Sen, A. (2004) Health Achievement and Equity: External and Internal Perspectives. In: Anand, S., Peter, F. and Sen, A. (eds) *Public Health, Ethics, and Equity*. Oxford: Oxford University Press, 263–268.

Siconolfi, D. E., Halkitis, P. N. and Moeller, R. W. (2015) Homo economicus: Young gay and bisexual men and the new public health. *Critical Public Health* 25, 554–568.

Singh, P. (2016) *Dying and Living in the Neighborhood: A Street-Level View of America's Healthcare Promise*. Baltimore, MD: Johns Hopkins University Press.

Solomon, M. (2015) *Making Medical Knowledge*. New York: Oxford University Press.

Soranno, P. A., Cheruvelil, K. S., Elliott, K. C. and Montgomery, G. M. (2015) It's good to share: Why environmental scientists' ethics are out of date. *BioScience* 65, 69–73.

Ståhl, T., Wismar, M., Ollila, E., et al. (2006) *Health in All Policies: Prospects and Potentials*. Finland: Finnish Ministry of Social Affairs and Health.

The Lancet Editors. (1994) Population health looking upstream. *The Lancet* 343, 429–432.

Torres, S., Labonté, R., Spitzer, D. L., et al. (2014) Improving health equity: The promising role of community health workers in Canada. *Healthcare Policy* 10, 73–85.

Welch, V. A., Akl, E. A., Guyatt, G., et al. (2017) GRADE Equity guidelines 1: Health equity in guideline development-introduction and rationale. *Journal of Clinical Epidemiology* 90, 59–67.

World Health Organization. (1986) Ottawa Charter for Health Promotion. Ottawa, ON: World Health Organization.

World Health Organization. (2015) Health in All Policies Training Manual. Geneva: World Health Organization.

Index

Page numbers in **bold** denote tables, those in *italics* denote figures.